W9-BZV-601

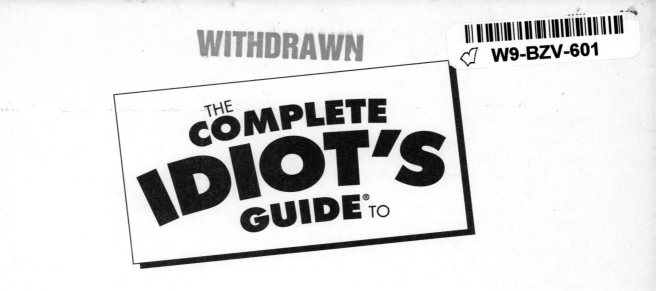

THE COMPLETE IDIOT'S GUIDE® TO

Bipolar Disorder

by Jay Carter, Psy.D., and Bobbi Dempsy

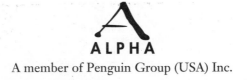

ALPHA

A member of Penguin Group (USA) Inc.

Dedicated to Julie Fast.

ALPHA BOOKS

Published by the Penguin Group

Penguin Group (USA) Inc., 375 Hudson Street, New York, New York 10014, USA

Penguin Group (Canada), 90 Eglinton Avenue East, Suite 700, Toronto, Ontario M4P 2Y3, Canada (a division of Pearson Penguin Canada Inc.)

Penguin Books Ltd., 80 Strand, London WC2R 0RL, England

Penguin Ireland, 25 St. Stephen's Green, Dublin 2, Ireland (a division of Penguin Books Ltd.)

Penguin Group (Australia), 250 Camberwell Road, Camberwell, Victoria 3124, Australia (a division of Pearson Australia Group Pty. Ltd.)

Penguin Books India Pvt. Ltd., 11 Community Centre, Panchsheel Park, New Delhi—110 017, India

Penguin Group (NZ), 67 Apollo Drive, Rosedale, North Shore, Auckland 1311, New Zealand (a division of Pearson New Zealand Ltd.)

Penguin Books (South Africa) (Pty.) Ltd., 24 Sturdee Avenue, Rosebank, Johannesburg 2196, South Africa

Penguin Books Ltd., Registered Offices: 80 Strand, London WC2R 0RL, England

Copyright © 2009 by Jay Carter and Bobbi Dempsey

International Standard Book Number: 978-1-59257-817-7
Library of Congress Catalog Card Number: 2008937764

11   10   8   7   6   5   4   3   2

Interpretation of the printing code: The rightmost number of the first series of numbers is the year of the book's printing; the rightmost number of the second series of numbers is the number of the book's printing. For example, a printing code of 09-1 shows that the first printing occurred in 2009.

Printed in the United States of America

Note: This publication contains the opinions and ideas of its authors. It is intended to provide helpful and informative material on the subject matter covered. It is sold with the understanding that the authors and publisher are not engaged in rendering professional services in the book. If the reader requires personal assistance or advice, a competent professional should be consulted.

The authors and publisher specifically disclaim any responsibility for any liability, loss, or risk, personal or otherwise, which is incurred as a consequence, directly or indirectly, of the use and application of any of the contents of this book.

Most Alpha books are available at special quantity discounts for bulk purchases for sales promotions, premiums, fundraising, or educational use. Special books, or book excerpts, can also be created to fit specific needs.

For details, write: Special Markets, Alpha Books, 375 Hudson Street, New York, NY 10014.

Publisher: *Marie Butler-Knight*
Editorial Director/Acquiring Editor: *Mike Sanders*
Senior Managing Editor: *Billy Fields*
Senior Development Editor: *Phil Kitchel*
Production Editor: *Kayla Dugger*

Copy Editor: *Teresa Elsey*
Cover Designer: *Kurt Owens*
Book Designer: *Trina Wurst*
Indexer: *Angie Bess*
Layout: *Chad Dressler*
Proofreader: *Mary Hunt*

Contents at a Glance

Contents

Introduction

Bipolar disorder affects more people than you might think. Sure, there are more than 5 million Americans who actually have the condition. But there are also the relatives, friends, coworkers, and other acquaintances of all of those bipolar people. As you probably already know very well, bipolar disorder doesn't just affect the person who actually has BP—it also affects everyone around the person, sometimes in a major way.

If you've been diagnosed with BP recently, you may have lots of questions and concerns. We hope this book will answer most (if not all) of them for you.

Even if it's been a while since your diagnosis, there may still be things about BP that confuse or challenge you. Once again, we hope this book will prove helpful to you in solving some of those bipolar riddles.

We would also suggest sharing this book with loved ones. (Better yet, get them copies of their own—it makes a great gift!) Once they have a better understanding of the disorder and what it's like to live with it every day, they may have a newfound sympathy and compassion for your daily struggles. They may also realize that many of your behaviors and actions are caused by your disorder, and aren't anything personal.

In the end, we hope you find this book informative, educational, and maybe even a little inspiring.

What You'll Find in This Book

This book is designed to be easily understood by the average person—someone who has bipolar disorder (or knows someone who does) but isn't a medical or psychiatric expert. With that in mind, we try to keep things as basic and jargon-free as possible. In certain sections, you will find some official or medical terms, simply because those are necessary to provide a proper explanation. However, we've made a concentrated effort to explain those big terms in an easy-to-understand way.

If you lose your place or forget where a particular topic was covered, there's a wonderfully comprehensive and detailed group of contents pages, so you can easily locate everything in a snap.

To make things even easier, the chapters have been organized into five separate parts:

In **Part 1, "Bipolar Disorder Basics,"** we cover (you guessed it) all of the basic stuff, like what exactly bipolar disorder is and how it happens. We separate fact from fiction, and clarify how BP differs from other conditions for which it is sometimes mistaken. We also cover the important issues of diagnosis and dual diagnoses in this part.

In **Part 2, "Symptoms/Effects of Bipolar Disorder,"** we discuss all of the signs and symptoms associated with BP. We start off with the two biggies—manic episodes and depression—and also cover some of the lesser-known symptoms. We tell you how to know when things are getting serious, and what to do about it. Lastly, we address the specific issues faced by young people who have bipolar disorder.

In **Part 3, "Treatment,"** we discuss the various treatment options available to help you handle your bipolar disorder. We start off by explaining why you need a treatment plan and how to organize one. We then delve into the actual treatment options, and alert you to their pros and cons. Lastly, we talk about hospitalization and what you need to know should you (or a loved one) ever need to be hospitalized for a BP-related problem.

In **Part 4, "Living With Bipolar Disorder,"** we shed some light on what it's really like to live with this condition 24/7. This may be familiar territory to many of you, especially if you were diagnosed a while ago. But you just might learn a few new things—and it may be very helpful to share this section with loved ones, so they can get a better understanding of your daily reality.

In **Part 5, "For Families,"** we include lots of information that will be helpful to your friends and loved ones. We hope you will encourage them to check out this section.

That's not all, though. Following those chapters, we include two more "bonus" elements. Appendix A is a glossary of important terms related to bipolar disorder. Appendix B is full of BP-related resources, including support groups and organizations that can help you learn more about this condition.

Extras

In addition to the main narrative of *The Complete Idiot's Guide to Bipolar Disorder,* you'll find other useful types of information. Here's how to recognize these features:

def•i•ni•tion

Sometimes it can seem as if BP has a language of its own. These sidebars will provide helpful definitions of many terms included in this book.

Mental Note

These sidebars provide helpful tips and little nuggets of information related to bipolar disorder.

Red Flag

When it comes to bipolar disorder, there are many serious issues you need to know about. These sidebars alert you to an important warning.

Real People

We think it's important for you to hear from other people who have bipolar disorder, in their own words. These sidebars contain firsthand accounts from bipolar people.

Research Says

These sidebars contain statistics, research findings, and other data compiled from studies and surveys related to bipolar disorder.

Acknowledgments

Thanks to my lovely wife for putting up with yet another book. Thanks to the brilliant and lovely Rita Warner, M.S. Thanks to Dr. Jon Gransee, Mavis Humes, Dr. David O'Connell, Robert Anthony, Verena Cole, Patricia C. Friel, M.S., and BP Extraordinaire (wherever you are). Thanks to my personable, patient agent Marilyn Allen of Allen O'Shea Literary Agency, Nikki Chong, Nancy Blaha, Jeff Young, Sandra Young, and Jessica Erkert. Thanks to my daughter, Shannon, and my son, JR. Thanks to Shannon Martinez, Jeff Carter, Patty Carter M.A., my readers, anonymous contributors, and my special seminar attendees. Thanks to my special BP mom, Pearl Carter-Gutkoski, who gave me life, and father, Mark Taylor Carter, who helped give me life. Thanks to the dedicated Dr. Kiki Chang, Cross Country Education, Hannah, my friend Barbara K-S, Lynn Shaw, the closet BPs, the dedicated BP researchers and mentors, DBSA, NAMI, NIMH, and all the people who have contributed but have slipped my mind for the moment. A *very* special thanks to Julie Fast who made this book possible. —Dr. Jay Carter

Bobbi Dempsey wishes to acknowledge her beloved grandmother, Bernice Kane, who passed away as this book was being written. She was loved by many and will be deeply missed.

Part 1

Bipolar Disorder Basics

We figured it made sense to start this book at the beginning, so in this part, we'll cover all of the basic information about bipolar disorder. If you are newly diagnosed, much of this material will be new (and hopefully helpful). But even old veterans will probably learn a thing or two.

About Bipolar Disorder

In This Chapter

- ◆ Bipolar disorder, by the numbers
- ◆ Tracing the roots of BP
- ◆ Understanding BP's cyclical nature

We have lots of information about bipolar disorder to share, but in this chapter we'll start with the basics. You'll learn what bipolar disorder is, how it manifests itself, and just how many people have it. We'll also address some myths and misconceptions about the condition.

Bipolar Stats

Just how common is bipolar disorder (BP)? It affects more people than you might think. The National Institute of Mental Health estimates that about 5.7 million American adults (or about 2.6 percent of the adult population) have the condition. However, it's possible that many more suffer from BP but have been misdiagnosed or are undiagnosed.

This underreporting of bipolar disorder happens for several reasons. For one thing, the remaining stigma attached to mental illness makes many people reluctant to admit they may have a problem or to seek treatment.

Instead, they may try to self-medicate. Many who self-medicate use alcohol, so some people thought of as alcoholics may actually have bipolar disorder or a subdromal form of bipolar disorder. A subdromal form causes mood swings, lack of sleep, racing thoughts, and talkativeness, but, because the level or severity of these symptoms falls beneath the diagnostic criteria for bipolar disorder, BP can not technically be diagnosed. The popular term for this is "soft bipolar." But these people can still be helped with treatments more effective than self-medicating.

The symptoms of bipolar disorder can look a lot like the symptoms caused by other disorders, making a concrete diagnosis difficult. One of the most consistent things about bipolar disorder is that it can be inconsistent. People with bipolar disorder may also have one or more other physical or mental conditions, and they may receive treatment only for one problem. Or another problem may mask the patient's bipolar symptoms. Bipolar disorder may start with only one symptom and slowly emerge until it finally has enough symptoms to be diagnosed.

Last, many medical professionals—especially general-practice MDs—don't have the specialized training required to accurately diagnose BP. This can be especially problematic in parts of the country (or the world) where there aren't enough specialists to evaluate possible cases of bipolar disorder. Currently, only 6 percent of family doctors are trained to treat bipolar disorder. There is a greater need for family doctors to intervene, as it is starting to be seen as less of a psychiatric problem and more of a physiological problem, like diabetes. A diabetic could be diagnosed with a personality disorder if they are having low blood sugar, but they do not have a personality disorder. The same is true for bipolar disorder, where the dopamine centers in the brain cause a person to act abnormally, but when the brain chemicals are normalized with medication, they do not act that way.

Mental Note

Bipolar disorder strikes men and women in about equal numbers, and it affects people of all races, nationalities, and ethnic backgrounds.

History of Bipolar Disorder

Descriptions of bipolar disorder go all the way back to ancient Greece. The connection between depression and mania was noted in French psychiatrist Jean-Pierre Falret's eighteenth-century concept of circular madness with lucid (normal mood) intervals.

At the turn of the nineteenth century, German psychiatrist Emil Kraepelin established *manic-depression* as a term for a specific disease, mainly by showing it ran in families. He also introduced the *mixed state*, in which symptoms of both mania and depression coincide. He and his students further classified the illness and are responsible for the spectrum concept we use today.

The modern concept of bipolar disorder is said to have originated in the 1960s, in three independent monographs by Carl Perris, Jules Angst, and George Winokur.

Until recently, bipolar was called manic-depression, and both terms are still used interchangeably in many publications. The verifying discovery that manic-depression truly had a genetic basis gave it more medical legitimacy, so the new and improved

Mental Note _____

In the twentieth century, John Cade discovered that lithium carbonate was a successful treatment for bipolar. This was the first discovery of any substance that successfully treated a psychiatric condition.

term *bipolar disorder* was born to suit it. The term came into popular use in the 1980s and replaced manic-depressive disorder as a diagnostic term found in the *Diagnostic and Statistical Manual of Mental Disorders* (DSM).

What Is Bipolar Disorder?

Before we go any further, it would be helpful to define bipolar disorder. You may already be very familiar with the condition, but to make sure we're all on the same page, let's put it in concrete terms.

The Spectrum Defined

Autism, fetal alcohol syndrome, and bipolar are considered to be *spectrum disorders*. The severity of a spectrum disorder can run the gamut. You can have a slight case or a full-blown version. Where on the spectrum a case falls is based on the degree or severity of symptoms exhibited by the patient.

Many mental illnesses fall on a spectrum. We all get the blues or occasionally say something before thinking it through, but some of us live outside of the healthy range of human emotion. Depending on where your symptoms fall, you may have a "cool," mild case of bipolar or a "red-hot" case. It all depends on how unmanageable your life becomes.

You may also hear that bipolar is a mood disorder. While true, a better description is that bipolar at the full-blown end of its spectrum appears to be a mental, emotional, and behavioral disorder. It is still technically classified as a mental disorder because the sufferer may lose touch with reality. That classification may change, but it's an emotional disorder because the sufferer may feel too happy or too sad in response to a particular situation or experience those feelings for too long. And it's a behavioral disorder when actions based on extreme emotions may become dangerous or harmful to the sufferer or others.

Bipolar was originally called cyclothymic personality disorder. The term *cyclothymic* by itself refers to a very mild version of bipolar disorder characterized by mood swings. Bipolar disorder was never a personality disorder. It was likely classified as a personality disorder because of the ego, arrogance, and entitlement one sees in the mania. These are symptoms of mania and tell you nothing about the true personality of the individual.

Mental Note _____

The terms *unipolar* and *bipolar* were coined by Karl Kleist in 1953. Bipolar disorders are circular disorders, with episodes of both mania and depression and *cycloid psychoses*, a term used for psychoses that are separate from both schizophrenia and affective psychoses. The psychosis of bipolar disorder usually comes as a secondary result of the loss of sleep, which is caused by the mania.

The spectrum of bipolar disorder ranges from the fringe of normal personality and temperament to full-blown impairment. When emotions and behaviors extend beyond the "fringe," thereby creating serious problems and dangerous behaviors, they can be considered a disorder. Those who suffer from "soft" or mild cases of bipolar, in contrast, may never need medication and may function without help.

Groups of symptoms that occur together are called *episodes*, *states*, or *phases*. A sufferer will be described as experiencing one of the following: mania, hypomania, depression, depressive mixed state, or mixed mania. Bipolar people are different from "normal" people in the number and severity of the symptoms involved in their episodes, as well as the duration of the episodes. Bipolar disorder magnifies normal emotions.

Type I and II

Bipolar is divided into subtypes based on the frequency, duration, and type of episodes a person experiences. To be diagnosed Bipolar I, you must manifest manic episodes, with or without a major depressive episode before or after. Either way, the episodes (with severe lack of sleep or severe chemical imbalance) can escalate into a psychotic expression, in which you lose touch with reality. This doesn't necessarily mean acting "crazy," per se, but rather that emotions may be magnified so much, for example, that the smallest annoyance can trigger shouting and rage, far outside any reaction that would be considered "normal."

In order to be diagnosed with Bipolar I, a patient must experience at least one instance of a specific period of abnormal (for the patient) persistent euphoria, agitation, irritability, or anger. This is usually followed by depression or suicidal despair. The patient may have also experienced hallucinations and/or delusions (from lack of sleep or chemical imbalance).

Red Flag

Psychosis and mania are the main factors that separate type I and type II. The symptoms of mania (defining Bipolar I) and hypomania (defining Bipolar II) are similar, apart from the presence of psychosis in mania. Psychotic mania is more severe and may require hospitalization. Some professionals say there is not a clear definition of I and II, and these subcategories may be changed in the newest DSM, scheduled to be published in 2012.

Psychosis and mania may be the criteria for some diagnosticians, but it can be unclear and can lead to misclassification. The lack of sleep may be the actual reason for psychosis. Bipolar mania cuts off the communication between the body and brain that says, "I need some sleep!" Hypomania may actually increase functioning, which may make the distinction between mania and hypomania somewhat clearer to you.

The spectrum disorder is not clearly defined in the DSM-IV. It is odd that the disorder is now recognized as a medical disorder, but the same subcategories were kept from when it was called "manic-depression." In the DSM-V, which is due out in 2012, there may be a more specific subcategorization. The DSM-V will contain updated diagnostic information based on the newest research. Two subcategories are helpful: bipolar with agitation and bipolar without agitation. These two subcategories correlate with the research on bipolar disorder with anxiety and bipolar disorder without anxiety. The research on "anxiety" may be actually referring to the agitation. Agitation may feel the same as anxiety, but if a person has bipolar disorder, it is more likely to be agitation than anxiety, which is medically different and treated differently.

Mental Note _____

As noted previously, the DSM is the *Diagnostic and Statistical Manual of Mental Disorders*. Published by the American Psychiatric Association, the guide has gone through several updated versions (designated by the number in Roman numeral that appears after DSM). Each new version of the DSM is more comprehensive, including new terms and conditions and often expanding on information about conditions previously listed.

These subcategories more clearly indicate the class of medication the sufferer should be prescribed and may be more helpful to physicians.

Bipolar II is usually marked by recurrent, major depressive episodes, either before or after a hypomanic episode. Type II is probably the more common type of bipolar.

The antidepressant-induced hypomania is currently considered Bipolar III and the rapid cycling is considered Bipolar IV. Rapid-cycling bipolar patients must have had at least four episodes (mania/hypomania and major depression) per year. Most rapid-cycling bipolar sufferers are Bipolar II patients. The anti-depressants called SSRIs (serotonin reuptakes) and tricyclics are the most notorious for causing mania. The current theory is that a person who develops mania from these medications must have the bipolar genetics. This author acknowledges that is usually true, but it may not be true in all cases. This author has seen a few cases of mania caused by medication when there was no evidence of bipolar disorder in the family genetics.

Mental Note _____

What's the difference between a disease and a disorder? According to Roget's Thesaurus and the Merriam-Webster and American Heritage dictionaries, *mental disease* and *mental disorder* are synonyms for the term *mental illness,* which seems to be the preferred term. So the answer is, not much, but you can catch a disease and cannot catch a disorder. Again, there is some controversy as to whether BP is a psychiatric or physiological illness.

Understanding Cycles

We all know that what goes up must come down. Of course, Newton was referring to gravity, but bipolar disorder takes a similar course, with the skyrocketing highs of euphoria (happiness) followed by the plummeting lows of melancholia (sadness) and sometimes irritability, anxiety (agitation), and rage in between. We describe this inevitable and drastic change in mood as a *cycle*.

Mania and Hypomania

The word *maniac*, from *mania* (Greek *maniakos*), means "lunatic" or "madman." People experiencing hypomania in ancient times might have been called lunatics, but that same behavior today, when accompanied by productivity, might be admired. Such great ideas in so little time! An executive with enough subordinates to carry out these ideas would be called brilliant. A one-man show who never actually carried out these ideas might be called an intellectual. And if you add an obsession to the mania, you might get a one-man show who could carry out his ideas—and we are back to brilliant. Eventually, however, the same thing happens to all brilliantly manic people: they crash (fatigue, depression). What goes up …

Manic phases can seem "happy" (as if you are really excited or hyper), or they can just make you feel anxious and irritated. The biggest problem caused by mania is the feeling of invincibility and superiority. This feeling is intoxicating and produces fearlessness, which contributes to poor decision-making and causes people to engage in extreme and risky behaviors. Many people with bipolar disorder have periods of delusions of grandeur (not necessarily psychotic) and believe they can do and get whatever they want. They think rules are for everyone else and do not apply to them. When we encounter such people, we call them egotistical, arrogant, or entitled.

def•i•ni•tion

> **Mania** is ungovernable enthusiasm. A **maniac** is someone with an inordinate or ungovernable enthusiasm for something.

Red Flag

> During a manic phase, a person will often act recklessly and exhibit little or no impulse control. This may be because the person feels invincible and may have delusions of grandeur, even to the point of thinking he or she is immortal. It also happens because they are unable to imagine the consequences of what they are doing.

Often a manic phase will last for days, preventing a person from sleeping. A few days with little or no sleep sets the stage for psychotic episodes. Obviously, losing touch with reality can be especially dangerous. Recklessness and a lack of fear of consequences do not always come with a good mood. Mania dominated by anger, irritability, and frustration can be very unpleasant for the sufferer, as well as for those around him or her. Episodes dominated by an ill-tempered mood ruin relationships when the sufferer makes cutting remarks or shows aggressive, violent behavior. These states often make the sufferer feel trapped, goaded, and out of control.

The Flip Side to Mania

Many bipolar people are very charismatic when they feel well and are able to entertain and manipulate others. Positivity and optimism are contagious. Many great and not-so-great leaders in world history are believed to have suffered from the disorder.

Most times, however, a high flyer will plummet and crash into a depressed state. The sufferer may sleep for 12 to 14 hours a day and feel empty and void while he or she is awake. The sufferer may have suicidal thoughts. The low can feel just as intense as the high he or she fell from. It's also a major disappointment after such exuberance. This Jekyll-to-Hyde transition is often blamed for a higher suicide rate among those with bipolar than those with other mental illnesses. People with unipolar depression cannot miss the highs they never had.

Untreated symptoms of mania and hypomania can last up to three months. Symptoms include the following:

- Aggressive, provocative, and intrusive behavior
- Belief in exaggerated abilities
- Insomnia
- Substance abuse
- Being easily irritated and/or distracted
- Feeling extremely "high" or euphoric
- Hyperactivity
- Racing thoughts and rapid or pressured speech
- Poor judgment and reckless behaviors
- Hypersexuality

Clinical Depression

We have all felt depressed. How do you know whether you are just sad or if you have clinical depression?

Depression is considered a medical problem when nothing bad has happened, but you feel way down in the dumps, or when something bad happens and you feel sad or angry for much longer than normal. It is perfectly natural to feel bad and depressed after grief or a loss of some kind. It is not natural or healthy to feel hopeless for no reason or to stay hopeless without any relief for too long a time. Time is essential. Time heals, as they say. Every day after a loss should get just a tiny bit easier.

After a manic episode, people with bipolar disorder commonly experience a depressive episode. Symptoms of depression include the following:

- Anxiety or impending feelings of doom
- Feelings of guilt, hopelessness, worthlessness, or helplessness
- Inability to concentrate, remember, or make decisions
- Irritability
- Lack of appetite and weight loss, or increased appetite and weight gain
- Lack of interest or pleasure in usual activities, including sex
- Loss of energy
- Sadness and crying
- Hypersomnia
- Thoughts of suicide

Mixed States

A mixed state contains components of depression and mania. For instance, a bipolar person may feel the racing thoughts and boundless energy of mania but the sadness and worthlessness of depression. This combination of symptoms can lead to particularly dangerous behaviors, mainly because the sufferer feels bad, desperate, hopeless, and empty—yet full of energy and compelled to action.

Exciting activities may become irresistible due to the probability that some relief may come from them. When the desperation becomes overwhelming, anonymous and unprotected sex, illicit drug use, expensive shopping sprees, and gambling are activities that often appeal to people in a bipolar state. If the fear of contracting a disease or becoming pregnant from unprotected sex is less powerful than the urge to feel close, loved, and wanted—even in less than ideal circumstances—the latter will win out.

> **Real People**
>
> A person with bipolar disorder who was having a long-running manic episode said, "I feel so exhausted ... and so energized."

Also, the intensity of an emotion, in this case hypersexuality, is exponentially greater in a bipolar person than in a healthy person.

Meanwhile, the proper feelings of fear and restraint are muted. Perhaps worst of all, the temporary ego/arrogance may encourage the person to think they are special, and therefore not susceptible to disease or injury. It is this emotional detachment from how their behaviors will affect them that can cause serious trouble.

Bipolar Myths and Misconceptions

Many things about bipolar are commonly misunderstood or misconstrued. Let's address a few of the most common misconceptions.

Myth #1: Mental disorders aren't real illnesses. False! Mental disorders are real illnesses. Bipolar is a real, chronic episodical illness and requires treatment just like diabetes, arthritis, or asthma.

Myth #2: If you exercise enough self-discipline, you can prevent yourself from being incapacitated by a mental disorder. False! People with mental disorders may win a particular battle, but they are incapable of winning the war. Furthermore, why should we have to spend all our time fighting?

Myth# 3: No one recovers from mental illness. False! Many people stricken with mental illness were normal and healthy for years before they got sick. In the same respect, they can recover as suddenly as they fell ill. Alternatively, their illnesses can be treated or managed so successfully that episodes are temporary and may not return.

Myth #4: It is risky to hire people with mental disorders to do important jobs. False! As long as a person is aware of his or her problems and is being treated, there is no reason for such prejudice. In fact, many famous people are bipolar, and often people with the disorder are very intelligent, highly motivated, and successful in their endeavors.

Myth #5: Mentally ill people are dangerous. False! Most people with a mental disorder are not dangerous. When mentally ill people act violently, it is usually for the same reasons that healthy people act violently, such as excessive intoxication. Most bipolar people who behave dangerously are experiencing a mixed episode and abusing a substance when they lash out. They are much more likely to commit suicide than to kill another person. They are also more likely to be the victim of violence than the perpetrator.

What Bipolar Isn't

Mental disorders may share common symptoms. Misdiagnosis, as a result, is not uncommon. Bipolar disorder is often confused with other mental illnesses, including attention deficit hyperactivity disorder (ADHD), clinical depression, schizophrenia, and borderline personality disorder (BPD). It has often been mistaken for various physical problems, such as Cushing's disease, hypothyroidism, multiple sclerosis (MS), lupus, and temporal lobe epilepsy (TLE).

A blurry line exists between what we consider a "physical illness" and what constitutes a "mental illness." The categories can be somewhat arbitrary, rather than being based on any scientific reasoning. Diagnoses in the DSM are based on behavior. The cause of the behavior is not determined just because the behavior is labeled. A person with bipolar disorder, for example, can act like someone with a borderline personality disorder when the bipolar genetics get riled. But for the sake of abiding by mainstream terminology, we will maintain this contestable medical distinction.

Attention Deficit Hyperactivity Disorder (ADHD)

ADHD is a neurological behavioral disorder, which manifests as hyperactivity, distractibility, impulsivity, and forgetfulness. Onset is during childhood and less than half of those affected "grow out" of the condition by adulthood. The differences between ADHD adults and bipolar adults are rather obvious. With children, the two are more difficult to discern, but upon deeper examination, differences arise.

An ADHD child's tantrums may be set off by sensory overstimulation or not getting his way, and the tantrums usually last up to 20 minutes. A bipolar child's fits are set off by limit setting and tend to last much longer. Bipolar children are often depressed and/or irritable; ADHD children are not usually depressed. Bipolar children have night terrors and very realistic nightmares, often with vividly explicit gore; ADHD children do not. Bipolar children, often as early as preschool, begin danger-seeking behaviors, are grandiose (boastful) at times, have laughing fits, and experience sexual hyperawareness. ADHD children may engage in high-risk behaviors without realizing the dangers but are less prone to grandiosity, fits of laughter, and hypersexuality.

Clinical Depression

Clinical depression (unipolar depression) is a neurological chemical imbalance that may manifest as three or more of the following: bouts of prolonged sadness, crying spells, changes in appetite and sleep patterns, irritability, anger, worry, anxiety, pessimism, persistent lethargy, guilt, worthlessness, inability to concentrate, indecisiveness, loss of interest or indifference, social withdrawal, general malaise or fatigue, and recurring thoughts of death or suicide.

Clinical depression is often confused with bipolar disorder because most often the first symptoms of bipolar disorder are depressive. Bipolar II sufferers usually spend more time depressed than in manic or mixed states. They also represent the majority of bipolar cases. Unipolar depression differs only by the absence of mania and mixed states. The symptoms of bipolar depression and unipolar depression are otherwise indistinguishable to most.

Schizophrenia

Schizophrenia is a neurological disorder marked by social dysfunction and psychotic symptoms that last for at least six months. The psychotic symptoms exhibited must not stem from another mental illness or be traceable to illicit drug use, alcohol, or the side effects of medication. The subtype of bipolar easily confused with schizophrenia is Bipolar I, due to the symptoms of psychosis. A combination of substance abuse and severe insomnia accounts for the vast majority of psychotic episodes among bipolar patients.

After a person has lost sleep due to mania and/or had his brain chemistry severely unbalanced, he may show very similar signs to schizophrenia. Most mental health professionals would be unable to tell the difference until they took a history and were able to identify the source of the behavior. Remember, the descriptions in the DSM are descriptions of behavior. If someone walks in off the street, it may be hard to tell if they are at the end of their bipolar mania, or schizophrenic, or did too much crack, or have an organic brain problem. Schizophrenia is rare, affecting less than 1 percent of the U.S. population (about two million people). It is reportedly the mental illness most misunderstood by the public. Split personality is not a symptom of schizophrenia, and violent behavior is very unusual.

The term *psychotic*, despite its common use in depicting murderous madmen, merely means being unable to distinguish real from imaginary stimuli and inner thoughts from outside voices. Most dangerous schizophrenics commit violent acts years before the onset of their disease, which on average occurs around 25 years of age. There is a big difference between criminality and mental illness. Most schizophrenics wouldn't hurt a flea. A few schizophrenics are criminals and may act out their criminal nature. Those schizophrenics need to go to jail and without blaming their mental problems. It is rare that their mental health problem is the cause of a criminal act.

Schizotypal affective disorder is essentially a less severe form of schizophrenia, marked by extreme social anxiety and unusual speech patterns and habits.

Borderline Personality Disorder (BPD)

BPD is a recently defined illness. Some professionals contest the legitimacy of this disorder being separate from bipolar disorder. The latest explanation of the difference is that bipolar is a chemically based dysfunction, whereas borderline personality disorder is psychologically based. More evidence suggests that BPD is temperament based and is set off by post-traumatic stress disorder (often caused by sexual abuse).

The many symptomatic similarities with bipolar disorder include extreme mood episodes, impulsivity, and recklessness. Some of the distinguishing characteristics of BPD are that sufferers have a higher likelihood of self-mutilation or self-hatred, a history of unstable personal relationships, and a history of having been abused and/or neglected as children. Although people with bipolar disorder may cut themselves or have unstable relationships, they may not have a history of being sexually abused.

The bipolar disorder is seen as "hardware" (medication fixes it), whereas the borderline is seen as "software" (medication may help, but won't fix it). Need I remind you again that our diagnoses are based on behavior? It may be pretty difficult to tell the difference between someone with exacerbated bipolar behavior versus someone who has borderline personality disorder.

Cushing's Disease and Cushing's Syndrome

Also known as hypercortisolism, these are endocrine (glandular) disorders caused by high levels of cortisol (a hormone) in the blood. The disease and the syndrome have different root causes, but both result in elevated cortisol levels. A variety of problems, such as a tumor on your pituitary gland, a certain type of lung cancer, or steroid use (to treat inflammatory diseases such as arthritis, lupus, or asthma), can cause the adrenal gland (near the kidneys) to release too much cortisol in response to ACTH (a neurotransmitter) being released from the pituitary gland (in your brain).

Cortisol helps regulate your blood pressure; prepares the body to respond to danger; and regulates the way you convert proteins, carbohydrates, and fats into energy. Cushing's disease and syndrome are fairly rare, affecting about 15 people out of every million. People with these diseases can exhibit euphoria, depression, and psychosis.

Hypothyroidism or Hyperthyroidism

Your thyroid gland is located in your throat. Thyroid hormones mainly regulate your body's metabolism. An underproduction of thyroid hormones slows down your metabolism, causing lethargy, fatigue, depressive moods, memory loss, and irritability. The condition is common, causing five million people per year in the United States to seek treatment. Many people, especially women, have some degree of thyroid malfunction and don't know it. Some reports estimate that 10 percent of women have some degree of thyroid hormone deficiency.

Hyperthyroid (overproduction of thyroid hormones) can appear to look like mania. Younger children or adolescents are more prone to have this condition than adults.

Anyone who believes they suffer from a mental illness because of the aforementioned symptoms is advised to have a blood test to rule out hypothyroidism before beginning treatment for depression, bipolar, or any other mental dysfunction.

Multiple Sclerosis (MS)

MS is an autoimmune disease that affects the central nervous system. Specifically, antibodies mistakenly attack areas of the brain and spinal cord known as white matter. These are circuits of nerve cells that carry signals between the gray matter areas, where the processing is done. MS destroys the type of glial cells (oligodendrocytes) that produce a white insulation layer (myelin). Without the white fatty insulation layer, the electrical signals being carried by the nerve network are lost.

People with MS can exhibit depression or psychosis (3 percent), but its physical manifestations make it somewhat easier to spot. It is unlikely to be confused with bipolar disorder … as long as you know this.

The name *multiple sclerosis* refers to the scars left by the destruction of the white matter. Almost any neurological symptom can be caused by the disease, especially in its early stages. MS is estimated to afflict 300,000 people in the United States and two times as many women as men. Most sufferers experience their first symptoms between ages 20 and 40.

Lupus (Systemic Lupus Erythematosus)

According to some estimates, two million Americans have some form of lupus. Lupus is most common among minorities and women. Symptoms usually appear between ages 15 and 45. Lupus is a chronic autoimmune disease that can affect multiple organ systems, including the central nervous system.

Lupus is one of several diseases referred to as "the great imitators," because its symptoms vary widely depending on which organ systems are affected. When the central nervous system is affected, lupus often mimics other mental illnesses, including bipolar disorder. Sufferers commonly complain of persistent general malaise, joint pain, fatigue, memory loss, and confusion. The symptoms of lupus could be mistaken for depression, but it is not likely to be depression, except as a co-occurring symptom.

Temporal Lobe Epilepsy (TLE)

Epilepsy is a common chronic neurological disorder that manifests as recurrent seizures. These seizures are attributed to abnormal and excessive neuronal activity in the brain. There are several different epileptic syndromes that originate in different parts of the brain. One rare form, known as temporal lobe epilepsy (TLE), has been sometimes mistaken as mental illness. TLE seizures can start at almost any age. Sometimes the disorder is provoked, which means it begins following a head injury or an infection of the brain (such as meningitis), but other cases are unprovoked.

Seizures focused within the temporal lobes can vary widely in severity. A seizure may be so gentle the sufferer does not even notice its occurrence. Preceding these seizures, many people report intensely felt emotions and rich sensory experiences, such as vibrant colors. Oddly, memories of tastes, sights, smells, and various past experiences flooding into the consciousness are common just before the tremors hit. We are unable to find good statistics on how many people are affected by TLE.

One author who has worked in the prison system suggests that this disorder may be more common among people who have frequently used crack cocaine or methamphetamine.

Chronic Fatigue

If a person has been manic for three months and is only getting three hours of sleep a night, it will eventually take its toll. After the usual "crash," it is assumed that they have depression. Maybe, but it could just be chronic fatigue, or both depression and chronic fatigue. The only difference between chronic fatigue and depression is that with chronic fatigue, you want to do things—you just can't. With depression, you don't want to.

After mania or even during mania, when a person is put on medication, they assume the medication is making them tired and slow. Not necessarily! Few humans can tax their bodies for months with very little sleep without crashing for a period of time. Keep in mind that well-rested people may not have a problem with the medication making them tired or dull. It usually takes weeks (at least) to get over chronic fatigue. Consider the initial fatigue and slowness as part of recovery.

 Red Flag

Symptoms can be ambiguous and professionals can misdiagnose patients whose disorders they don't have much experience treating. It is extremely important that you provide a complete medical history to your doctor, regardless of her specialization. Writing down your symptoms before you see any physician is the best way to ensure you are not misunderstood and that you don't forget to say something relevant. Also probe your family history for disorders and write them down as well.

On the Horizon

There is good reason to be hopeful about the prognosis for people with bipolar disorder. Every day new discoveries are being made with regard to bipolar disorder, its treatment, and its causes.

Like diabetes, the disorder can be managed and regulated, but it cannot be cured. A regimen of psychotherapy, medication, diet, and exercise has so far proven to be the best treatment plan.

In the following chapters we will advise you on how to seek out the best doctor, therapist, and regimen for you. You must individualize your own treatment plan.

Whatever you do, don't give up on yourself! The feeling that comes from being liberated from your extreme moods and self-destructive behaviors is indescribably satisfying—we promise.

The Least You Need to Know

- ◆ It's difficult to pinpoint exact statistics related to bipolar disorder, since it's widely believed that many cases are undiagnosed or misdiagnosed.

- ◆ Bipolar disorder involves a succession of cycles, including manic phases followed by severe lows.

- ◆ Scientists and medical experts have made strides recently with regard to bipolar research, and there is reason to be optimistic about new developments on the horizon.

- ◆ Bipolar disorder can often be misdiagnosed or mistaken for another condition, so it's important for patients to be as detailed as possible when describing their symptoms.

- ◆ Bipolar medication is not to blame for a person feeling tired or crashing after taxing her body for a long period of time.

2

The Brain's Bipolar Perspective

In This Chapter

◆ A functional explanation of the mind

◆ Characteristics of the bipolar brain

◆ Examining the "chemical imbalance"

◆ How the bipolar brain makeup causes symptoms

To figure out how and why bipolar disorder happens, you need to understand the basics of how the brain works. Of course, the brain is a very complicated organ. But for the purposes of this chapter, we will try to make the explanation as simple as possible and give you a glimpse of how bipolar disorder affects the brain. We will begin with a functional explanation of the mind in simple terms. Bear with the explanation; the bipolar punch line is at the end of the explanation of the three mentalities.

To really help you understand the relationship between bipolar disorder and the brain, we analyze the brain from two different viewpoints. First, we'll discuss the psychological functions of the mind. Then we'll discuss the anatomical parts of the brain and how they function. Together, these two explanations should give you a pretty good vision of what goes on inside the head of someone with bipolar disorder.

First, we are going to dissect the mind (so to speak) into three psychological entities, in order to give you a practical explanation of how the brain is affected by bipolar disorder. After examining these three mentalities, we will take a look, from an anatomical perspective, at the psychological aspects of the brain and how they appear in a person with bipolar disorder.

The Mammal Mentality

Humans are born with what we'll call the "mammal brain." It operates on a stimulus-response, or cause-effect, basis. We associate one thing to a sound, or one behavior to a condition. We associate a one word command to an action. Your mammal operates under your command. You say "sit" and the mammal sits, except you don't have to say "sit," because your mammal brain automatically follows your internal commands.

The mammal carries the feelings of a person. During a depression, the mammal is the part that feels it. During mania, the mammal is the part that feels the euphoria, anger, or agitation. The limbic system of your brain is in the back of your brain and it is akin to what we call the mammalian brain, or mammal.

Pro-Survival vs. Anti-Survival

Some mammals have a stronger impulse for survival than others. Why does the mammal mentality run toward the chocolate? Because it has been programmed to. Mammals have been programmed for millions upon millions of years for one thing—survival. How are they programmed? They are programmed at the cellular level by Mother Nature. They are programmed that "pleasure is good" (pro-survival) and "pain is bad" (anti-survival). It is simple programming, and in the environment of Mother Nature, it works! If it feels good, it's probably good for you. If it doesn't feel good, it's probably not good for you. If it tastes good, eat it. If it doesn't taste good, don't eat it.

Without direction from the higher mentalities of the human being, the mammal would just do what it is programmed to do. In our society, however, there are things that feel good but are not good for you. Cocaine use may feel good, but it is not good for you. Consuming alcohol to excess is not good for you, and too much chocolate may not be good for you. But without the higher mentalities, the mammal snorts the cocaine, drinks the alcohol, and eats the chocolate. The mammal makes a good slave, but a very poor master. When the higher mentalities get lost in mania or depression, however, the mammal may be left to be the master.

Red Flag

The mammal mentality partially explains addiction. Our society offers things that feel good but are not necessarily good for you—like cocaine, alcohol, and (for some of us) chocolate. The mammal simply goes after the pleasurable activities. When the higher mentalities are lessened by mania, the ability to see consequences is less and the mammal has more reign. One of the symptoms of mania is doing things that are pleasurable with little regard for the consequences. That's one of the reasons that substance abuse occurs with bipolar disorder 60 percent of the time.

The Guard Dog at the Exit Door

The mammal can actually override your higher mentalities in moments where your survival is at stake. Let's say you decide that your life is over and you are going to jump off a bridge. You get a running start, but the mammal may stop you before you go over. Why? The mammal senses danger. It may not let you jump.

Did you ever almost fall asleep while driving, only to be suddenly jerked awake? That was the mammal. It senses danger. When a person gets to the edge of a bridge, the mammal may sense danger and say, "No way."

This overriding capability explains why I lie to myself when I reach for that bag of chocolates. I hear my cognitive area rationalizing and thinking, "I'll just have two." I know that's a lie, because in my entire life, I have never had just two chocolates. I have always endeavored to eat the whole bag, and I resentfully share it with my children if they catch me eating it. I hear myself rationalizing, "I'll exercise it off." I know that's a lie, because I never exercise.

Real People

A person with bipolar who had decided to jump off a bridge gave this explanation to an interviewer who asked, "Why didn't you jump?"

"I don't know. I wasn't looking for attention. I had truly decided to end it. Something stopped me. My body wouldn't jump. It just wouldn't."

The Cognitive Mentality

The cognitive area of the brain is believed to be no bigger than two walnuts. The cognitive area is fully formed at an early age—usually by age 7. It develops as we mature.

How can you tell when your cognitive ability was fully formed? Well, if you can remember when you were 3, that's when yours was formed. If you can't remember when you were 3, but you can remember first grade, it was fully formed by then.

Once the cognitive mentality is fully formed, we are capable of forming full sentences. Once we can form full sentences, we are capable of having rules and beliefs. Children operate on rules and beliefs. These rules and beliefs are downloaded into our cognitive mentality from our parents, school, church, television, peers, and so on. They form a concrete foundation for us to operate on. The cognitive mentality is not the highest mentality, as you will see later in this chapter. However, the rules and beliefs stored in the cognitive mentality are very important.

The cognitive part of your mind forms thoughts. When a person is manic and has racing thoughts, a second thought may interrupt a first thought before it is completed. Racing thoughts can be too fast and cause a lack of focus. A person in a state of mania thinks faster than others and may even get impatient with you if you don't talk fast enough. It is almost as if they exist in a different time continuum. When a person thinks so fast that he or she is totally consumed by the thoughts, we call it *catatonia*. It may not look like the person is doing anything, but the mind is spinning so fast, he or she can't even find time to perceive reality.

The cognitive "conscience" is based upon rules and beliefs. A child may not do a certain thing because "the minister says it's a sin," or because "Mom says I'll get hurt if I do that." The mammal has a conscience, too, based upon stimulus-response. It operates something like this: "I am not going to hit Johnny today, because I hit him yesterday—and he hit me back." We mention conscience because people in a manic state may be perceived to lack a conscience. We will later compare the cognitive and mammal consciences to the conscience of the highest mentality, the prefrontal lobe mentality, which is located in the front of your brain with the cognitive area just behind it.

The Prefrontal Lobe Mentality

Around the time we reach adolescence, our prefrontal lobe starts to come online. For some people, it develops later, and for others, it doesn't come online at all. We actually don't need a prefrontal lobe to function. If we have a good set of rules and beliefs, we can make it through this life okay without one.

The prefrontal lobe is a set of awarenesses. Our ability to have insight, foresight, and hindsight is housed in the lobe. Our ability to prioritize is in the lobe. We have self-awareness, the ability to weigh possible outcomes and benefit from our experience. Think of the prefrontal lobe as the captain's chair of your mind. The captain's chair sits on top of the ship and is surrounded with 360 degrees of windows, so the captain can see where he is going, where he has been, and what might be coming in from the sides.

Children and the Prefrontal Lobe

Children don't use their prefrontal lobes as much as adults do. Their prefrontal lobes have not matured yet. Children are not usually aware of their surroundings. A kid could be standing in front of a door that 50 people want to get through and be oblivious until someone finally says, "Hey kid, get out of the way!"

Seeing the Consequences

The prefrontal lobe is the part of you that visualizes the consequences of things you might be thinking about doing.

When people are manic, their prefrontal lobe goes out like a light bulb. That's why they may not exercise the best judgment during a manic phase. People who might normally be sensible can run up $20,000 of credit card debt, gamble away their life savings, have unprotected sex, or cheat on their spouses. They don't think about the consequences, because they can't. Their prefrontal lobe is off-line. They have no limits or boundaries, because limits and boundaries are set in context in the prefrontal lobe.

As you may already know, it's also pointless to try to argue with someone who is in a manic phase. When you're in this state, you are thinking six times faster than normal. You may be brilliant, but you have no judgment and no common sense. You don't see the consequences of your actions, because you can't.

Mental Note _____

If you suffer from bipolar disorder, make sure your loved ones know that your moods, outbursts, and other behaviors are not a personal attack on them, even when it might seem that way. It can help to remind them that these difficult periods are usually just temporary phases that will (eventually) go away.

Parts of the Brain

Okay, now that we've looked at your brain from a psychological perspective, let's switch gears and look at your brain from an anatomical viewpoint. Let's get to know the parts of the brain and the chemical messengers, called *neurotransmitters*, that generate electrical signals and make it function. Before we begin, here are two things to keep in mind:

First, most people find the Greek and Latin names used in neuroanatomy (the structure of the brain) hard to remember. To make matters worse, some parts of the brain have two or more names. We will try to provide the most common terms used today and to give their meanings in English. The literal meanings of neuroanatomy terms often refer to the shape or some other descriptive property of the structure they name, helping us identify them in real-life specimens. For example, amygdala means "almond," which refers to its shape. The amygdala is located at the basal part of your brain. A physical stimulus to the amygdala during brain operations causes anger, euphoria, or hypersexuality to the patient. These are all huge factors in bipolar disorder and the amygdala plays a large role in bipolar disorder.

Second, we want to stress that the following explanation of the brain's layout and function is very oversimplified. We will briefly explain the areas of the brain currently under investigation with respect to bipolar disorder. But keep in mind that, while the brain has centers that are specialized for specific tasks, these tasks can also be (and often are) performed by other areas of the brain, too. People with traumatic brain injuries, strokes, and diseases have "relearned" activities when other parts of the brain have taken over for areas lost or damaged.

Anatomically, the human brain can be divided into three main parts: the limbic system (mammal), the forebrain (prefrontal lobe and cognitive), and the hindbrain (dinosaur brain). Other anatomical elements like neurons, neurotransmitters, and hormones affect how the brain operates, so we will briefly touch on those in this chapter, as well.

The Limbic System

The limbic system, or middle brain, consists of the thalamus, hypothalamus, and amygdales. The limbic system is akin to the mammal part of your mind. As we said, when physically poked during a brain operation, the amygdala elicits euphoria, anger, or hypersexuality. Together, the parts of the limbic system monitor all of your internal organs and control your pituitary gland. They are the initial processing station for input coming from all of your senses. The pituitary gland is involved with our sleep rhythms. An interruption in sleep cycle is one of the significant triggers of mania. People with bipolar disorder are at risk to exacerbate their bipolar disorder when they work third shifts or swing shifts.

You don't decide to get hungry or sleepy or cold—you just suddenly feel that way. That is why the middle brain is nicknamed the "feed and breed" part of your brain.

The *thalamus*, or "marriage bed," is composed of two egg-shaped masses of nerve tissue, each of which is about the size of a walnut. The hypothalamus sits in front of and below the thalamus and is about a third of its size.

The amygdales are two almond-shaped groups of neurons located beneath the hypothalamus. Recently much research has been aimed at the amygdales. They have been the focus of many new discoveries, including that they give rise to emotional reactions and serve a role in emotional memory.

The Forebrain

The *cerebrum*, which actually means "brain," is the largest part of the forebrain. Just beneath its surface is, well, where you live inside your body. Some say the seat of the soul/spirit/consciousness is about 2 inches behind your eyes. The layer that lies just under the surface of the cerebrum is called the *cerebral cortex*. The cerebral cortex is the layer of the brain often referred to as gray matter.

The forebrain is the part of the brain that involves categorization of concrete and conscious experiences, feelings, and thoughts. It is the headquarters of emotions. It "sees" what you are feeling and decides whether to express that emotion or not. It is also the area that handles the concepts of rewards and consequences. Some studies of bipolar people have indicated a considerable inac-

Mental Note _____

The cortex is gray because nerves in this area lack the insulation that makes most other parts of the brain, like the limbic system, appear white.

tivity of gray matter in this area when they are experiencing symptoms, which may help explain why some people with BP have trouble grasping the consequences of their actions.

The forebrain is also the place where language is produced and understood. All of your voluntary movements and behaviors are here.

You might think of the limbic system as the brain's secretary or answering service. It logs all of the sensory information it receives, decides which is most important to the body's survival, and then passes that essential information along to the brain's command centers.

However, if the limbic system relays bad information, your forebrain will react in an inappropriate way. In other words, any miscommunication between your limbic system and your forebrain can lead to all sorts of problems, including inappropriate reactions and behaviors. If your cognitive brain is spinning with racing thoughts, and your prefrontal lobe is off-line, the limbic system only has the cognitive area to deal with, which can be cold and hyperrational. When the prefrontal lobe mentality is unable to set limits and boundaries for the limbic system, the cognitive area (always willing to help solve a problem) may take direction from the mammal to give the mammal what it wants.

The Hindbrain

The hindbrain is comprised of the brainstem and *cerebellum*, or "small brain." It is located just above your spine in the back of your head. Breathing and swallowing, two things you don't have to think about, are regulated by the brainstem. These are considered involuntary or "lower" mental functions.

You have two cerebellums, one on each side of the brainstem. Each of them is a small ball of neurons, and they are believed to coordinate your motor skills and complicated movements.

The hindbrain may play a role in bipolar disorder, but it is probably minor. Mania may in part come from the fight-or-flight response that begins in the brainstem. Fear or the anticipation of pain releases neurotransmitters and hormones that excite you or make you ready to act. These chemicals begin a complex physical response that readies you to either fight the threat or fly away from it, so to speak. These are considered lower involuntary mental functions or the "dinosaur" brain, which doesn't seem that involved in bipolar disorder. There may be some "loop" that takes place in the long temper tantrums noted with bipolar kids. It is speculated that the adrenaline and non-cathartic manic rage can form a seemingly endless loop, causing such long tantrums.

Neurons

The many areas and structures in the brain are wired together by long conga lines of neurons. The word *neuron* means "string" or "wire." Neurons consist of a cell body and two types of projections (dendrites and an axon). Some of the projections are wrapped in insulation called *myelin*.

The gaps between each neuron in the conga line are called *synapses* (meaning "to bind together"). Neurons communicate with each other at the synapses by sending electrical signals. These are changed into chemical signals or neurotransmitters, which travel across the synapse and become electrical signals again at the next neuron in the line. An improper balance of dopamine and other brain chemicals may deregulate the firing of this bio-electric system, causing bipolar symptoms.

The conga line has support all around it, called *glial cells*. Glial cells insulating the line and supporting it in a variety of functions. They can talk to neurons, who in turn can tell them what they need. Glial cells outnumber neurons about three to one in the central nervous system (the brain and spinal cord).

Neurotransmitters and Hormones

You may have heard that a person with mental problems has a "chemical imbalance." That is not entirely true most of the time; too much or too little of a neurotransmitter can cause communication problems in the brain. Too much of the neurotransmitter serotonin, for example, will make you ecstatic, and too little will make you depressed.

Serotonin is an example of an excitatory agent. As you can probably guess, excitatory agents make you happy or excited. But don't think you can drink a bunch of serotonin and be happy. That's like drinking 3 gallons of milk so you can grow 6 inches overnight. Doctors often prescribed *SSRIs* if a serotonin deficiency is suspected.

On the other side of the coin are inhibitory agents (such as melatonin) that help the body relax. For example, much melatonin is found in the body of a hibernating bear. An imbalance in these chemicals can throw your sleep routine out of whack, which is a common trigger for a bipolar episode.

def•i•ni•tion

SSRIs—selective serotonin reuptake inhibitors—are a commonly prescribed type of antidepressants, used to increase the levels of serotonin in the brain. Research as of this writing shows that these antidepressants are not effective in treating bipolar depression.

Brain Waves

One way to see what your brain is doing is to measure the amount and type of electricity it's producing. Yes, the chemicals in your brain produce electrical pulses important to communication between neurons. An EEG (electroencephalograph) chart recorder is painlessly wired to your head with sticky pads called electrodes. The chart shows the different kinds of brain waves you emit according to the state of affairs in your brain. These brain waves are very tiny electrical signals, just a few millionths of a volt.

Children mainly produce theta brain waves in their immature brains, which leads to their wild imaginations. Adults with mature brains mainly produce alpha and delta waves. Only severely disturbed adults mainly produce theta waves.

Brain waves originate from the forebrain's cerebral cortex, but they also reflect activities going on in other parts of the brain. Electrical changes are related directly to types of neuronal activity. Brain waves vary in strength and frequency, with a particular contrast between sleep and wakefulness. Beta brain waves are involved in higher mental activity, including perception and consciousness. Alpha brain waves are generated in the thalamus, while theta brain waves occur mainly in the cerebrum. Alpha and theta brain waves are linked with creative, insightful thought. Delta waves occur during sleep. In neuro-feedback sessions, a person with BP can be taught to reduce the importance of certain thoughts, as if learning to not listen to a radio playing in the background. Different brain waves can be measured and instructions given accordingly by the therapist.

Brain Development

The first three years of life are a period of incredible growth and development. At birth, your brain is about 25 percent of its approximate adult weight of 3 pounds. By age 3, your brain has grown dramatically, producing billions of cells (neurons and glia) and hundreds of trillions of connections, or synapses, between these cells. This explosion of growth in your forebrain includes the several lobes of the cerebral cortex. At that point, the brain is ready for complex mental functions such as thought, reason, and abstraction. A young child doesn't have the same abilities as an adult, but can still come up with some pretty witty stuff.

An adolescent of 15 has near-adult reasoning ability. This is especially true if you are female, as many males' brains do not mature until they are nearly 20. This is usually when the prefrontal lobe starts coming online. You start seeing the bigger picture (to some degree). You start becoming self-aware and therefore other-aware.

So why are teenagers so darn crazy? Hormones and neurotransmitters (and hormones that are also classified as neurotransmitters) are constantly barraging the adolescent brain. A person must become accustomed to these constant chemical cocktails over time.

Recent research suggests that teens use a different part of the brain than adults do to weigh risks and make judgments. Bipolar disorder often starts becoming more evident during adolescence. A teenager becomes asymptomatic or symptomatic as hormonal changes exacerbate BP. It can be tricky to diagnose BP at this age, partly because some BP behaviors—risk-taking and irregular sleep patterns, for example—are also commonly found in many non-bipolar teenagers.

Physical or Psychiatric?

So is bipolar disorder a mental condition or a physical condition? That's a good question. There has been (and to some extent still is) debate about whether to classify bipolar disorder as a physical or psychiatric condition.

Originally, bipolar disorder was called *cyclothymic personality disorder*. That term was probably based on the cyclical nature of the condition—as well as the (now outdated) belief that the typical bipolar behaviors were simply personality traits.

We now know this is not a personality disorder. The ego, arrogance, and entitlement one sees in bipolar disorder are symptoms of mania. It could also be the symptoms of being a jerk, so there must be other bipolar symptoms to make an accurate diagnosis. I will again caution you not to make any judgments about the personality of someone who does happen to be bipolar. (Not all people who have these traits are manic.) *Manic-depression* was the term coined for bipolar disorder in the recent past, and some people still use that term.

Once experts agreed that this condition was a medical disorder, *bipolar disorder* became the accepted term. It is not a psychological problem (although it may cause one), and it is not a personality problem (although it may affect personality).

The Benefits of a Broader Classification

There are some excellent benefits to the treatment of bipolar disorder as a physiological disorder, rather than a psychiatric disorder. First of all, it *is* a physiological disorder, so that's the most accurate approach.

From a practical standpoint, classifying bipolar as a physiological disorder may make it easier for patients to receive the treatment they need as quickly as possible. General practitioners can be trained to treat bipolar disorder as a physical illness. Of course, more complicated cases still have to be referred to a psychiatrist or to the ER.

> ⟩**Real People** _____
>
> Co-author Jay travels across the country giving seminars, and he hears many stories about the difficulties in treating bipolar disorder. For example, in California's Sonoma County, as of this writing, there are no psychiatric wards open. A person who needs treatment gets referred to San Francisco, which is over an hour away. This is why, if you have bipolar disorder, the best way to deal with it is prevention. Take your meds and be diligent about your other forms of treatment.

The Bipolar Brain vs. the Healthy Brain

Your brain is a biological organ like your heart or liver. Doctors and technicians use a special camera to take a picture of it. This is called a *SPECT* or SPET scan and it produces an image of what your brain is actually doing in there.

How a SPECT Test Works

A substance, called a *tracer*, that emits gamma rays is injected into the patient. The tracer travels to parts of the brain that need more blood—the parts that are most active. When the patient's brain is scanned, the tracer causes places with lots of activity to light up more than places with less activity. A really neat three-dimensional image is put together from all of the scans and voilà! We can see what the brain is doing and the relative sizes of the brain's different parts. In brains with disorders, some parts may be smaller than normal or less packed with neurons (less dense) than normal.

def•i•ni•tion _____

SPECT, which stands for single photon emission computed tomography, is used to see how blood flows through the arteries and veins in your brain.

What Will the Doctor See If I'm Bipolar?

Bipolar brains light up more in an area that processes emotions (the amygdales) and less in the area that regulates or suppresses emotions (the prefrontal cortex, or prefrontal lobe). They tend to have a normal number of neurons, but they're smaller, with fewer dendrites (projections) emanating from them. Dendrites reach out to other neurons and connect the brain's circuitry. The circuitry can get discombobulated (not a scientific term) when there's a chemical imbalance in the brain, causing some brain cells not to fire and others to fire too much.

In a disease like Alzheimer's, we see neuronal degeneration occur. The neurons literally wither and die. Bipolar brain cells do not show degeneration, except in cases of certain types of substance abuse. Whereas Alzheimer's, methamphetamine, cocaine, amphetamines, and so on actually kill brain cells, bipolar disorder does not. The cells are not firing, but they are not dead.

If a doctor performs a scan while you are manic, she will see hyperactivity in certain parts of your brain. Those parts will be lit up like a Christmas tree. On the other hand, if you are depressed when your brain is scanned, your brain may show hypoactivity, meaning the lights have become very dim on the Christmas tree.

The Least You Need to Know

- Many different parts of the brain play a role in bipolar disorder.
- During and after a manic episode, an affected person may lose insight, foresight, hindsight, context, and the ability to see himself or herself.
- People who are manic do not see the consequences of their actions.
- Originally deemed a personality disorder, bipolar disorder is now generally recognized as a medical condition.

Causes

In This Chapter

- ◆ The role of genetics
- ◆ Things that trigger bipolar episodes
- ◆ Environmental conditions

How exactly does bipolar disorder happen? Well, there are several possible explanations. We've already talked about the brain systems and chemicals that play a role. But other factors are also believed to cause or at least contribute to bipolar disorder. And still other things happen (trauma, hormone imbalances, drug use) that may look like causes of bipolar disorder, though they merely exacerbate bipolar episodes.

Bipolar disorder is genetic and chemical, but it almost always has to be exacerbated (stimulated) by something like hormones or trauma. In this chapter, we will discuss the preexisting genetics and some of those triggers.

Genetics

Statistics show that up to 3.2 percent of the population has bipolar disorder. In reality, there are more than 3.2 percent, because 20 to 40 percent of people who have the genetics to develop bipolar disorder never have it exacerbated and so never show symptoms. In twin studies, an identical twin has a 60 to 80 percent chance of having symptoms of bipolar disorder if the twin sibling has developed bipolar symptoms. To extrapolate from this, that must mean that 20 to 40 percent of people with bipolar genetics never have symptoms.

The latest finding in bipolar genetics is that a single gene accounts for 10 percent of people with bipolar disorder (GRK-3). Three other chromosomal regions are suspected. This means that there may be four different genes for bipolar disorder. We don't yet know for sure exactly which genes contribute to bipolar disorder, but we know other genes are involved. If there are four genes, then there are at least 16 different possible combinations of bipolar disorder. Some of these genes may be more dominant than others. In the United States, a child only has an 8 percent chance of having bipolar disorder if one parent has it. However, this author has seen families with five children where four have bipolar disorder, and seen families of five kids where none of them do.

GRK-3 has been found to cause hypersensitivity to dopamine, the major brain chemical involved in bipolar disorder. This affects the dopamine centers in the brain. The use of certain drugs, such as amphetamines, seems to affect the same dopamine centers that are affected by mania, so it's not surprising that manic behavior is often similar to the behavior of someone who has taken amphetamines. Psychostimulants like amphetamines, meth, and cocaine are thought to increase dopamine release, which can cause mania as well as mimic mania.

These behaviors can vary from one person to another, but often include the following:

- Thinking faster than normal
- Diminished executive functions (insight, foresight, hindsight)
- Diminished feelings (except for euphoria, anger, hypersexuality)
- Pupils look like pin points or dilated

These symptoms would all exemplify the GRK-3, chromosome 22, hypersensitivity to dopamine.

In the United States, if one parent has bipolar disorder, the children have an 8 percent chance of being diagnosed with the disorder. These odds are different in other countries, which means one of two things:

◆ People in other countries may be assessed for bipolar disorder differently than we assess here in the United States.

◆ There are slightly different bipolar genetics in certain parts of the world.

For example, in Switzerland, there is a 15 percent chance that the child of a parent with BP will be diagnosed with bipolar disorder. This shows that the way we diagnose bipolar disorder may vary from decade to decade and from country to country. It is definitely not a finite diagnosis, and at this point in our knowledge of bipolar disorder, it is primitive. At some point, we will be able to diagnose bipolar disorder with a genetic test. The test would be very helpful in families where bipolar disorder was rampant. That way, preventatives could be initiated for those who had the genetics. We are not there yet.

Mental Note _____

Studies of identical twins show that if one twin has bipolar disorder, the other twin has a 60 to 80 percent chance of exhibiting bipolar behavior. That is because environmental factors also play a role in the development of bipolar disorder vs. just having the genetics, and that could mean that 20 to 40 percent of people with the genetics that cause bipolar disorder never have an episode.

One also has to take into account that these are general statistics, which have not been broken down into specifics because we have not identified all the specific genes yet. If four different chromosomal regions appear to be factors for bipolar disorder, there must be many different combinations and types of bipolar disorder. We are not sure which of these genes may have a dominant or recessive quality.

Dr. Russell Barkley (the prominent expert on ADHD, currently a research professor in the Department of Psychiatry at the SUNY Upstate Medical University in Syracuse, New York) states that three genes contribute to ADHD. He believes designer drugs will be created for all of these combinations. If there are three genes, there are likely to be nine different designer drugs. If there are four genes for bipolar disorder, there may be 16 different designer drugs (combination-specific formulas) for bipolar disorder. We are not there yet, but with a little bit more funding and research, we could be there soon.

Bipolar disorder is a family illness. If bipolar disorder runs in your family and you didn't get the genetics, you are just lucky. Not having the disorder, however, doesn't mean you aren't affected. I don't know of any families in which someone's bipolar disorder doesn't affect the rest of the family in some way. Certain psychiatrists will not treat an individual for bipolar disorder. They insist on bringing the family and/or significant other into treatment, which seems to greatly improve the outcome.

A Bipolar "Thermometer"

You could look at BP like a thermometer. A thermometer measures degrees of heat. Bipolar disorder, being a spectrum disorder, also has degrees of symptoms. Let's suppose you have a bipolar thermometer with 10 degrees of intensity.

10: Bipolar I
 9: Bipolar II severe
 8: Bipolar II medium
 7: Bipolar II low
 6: Most traits—not diagnosable now
 5: More traits—not diagnosable now
 4: Some traits—not diagnosable now
 3: Most tendencies—never diagnosable
 2: More tendencies—never diagnosable
 1: Few tendencies—never diagnosable
 0: Temperament

If we look at the bigger picture of bipolar disorder, we know it gets triggered by things. If you are a 5 (which is not diagnosable) and you get severely traumatized, that could raise you to an 8 (which is diagnosable). Medication and EMDR (eye movement desensitization and reprocessing, a form of treatment for trauma) may bring you back to a 5 or 6.

If you are a 4 and go through a difficult menopause, that could raise you to a 7. Hormone balancing and medication may bring you back to a 4 or 5.

If you are a 6 and you binge or become dependent on drugs or alcohol, it could raise you to a 10 temporarily. Detoxing and medication may bring you down to a 3 or 4, if you stay on medication.

These are examples. They are not cast in stone. If you are Bipolar I, you may vacillate in the 6 to 10 range. If you are Bipolar II, you may vacillate in the 1 to 8 range. It depends on genetics, body chemistry, and events.

The worst combination for bipolar disorder is bipolar and hormones. You can see this in the fact that over 60 percent of people eventually diagnosed with bipolar disorder report that they had bipolar symptoms between the ages of 15 and 20 years old, when their hormones were overactive. The second worst combination seems to be bipolar and PTSD (post-traumatic stress disorder). If someone is a 5 on the scale, they are not diagnosable. But if that person gets traumatized, for example, in a military event, it may bump them up to an 8, which is diagnosable.

Can You "Become" Bipolar?

You may wonder if a person can "become" bipolar. The answer is no, although it may look that way. For example, a person may carry the genes for bipolar disorder throughout life and suddenly "become bipolar" in their elderly years. There are usually two explanations for this:

◆ The person may have been disrupted from his or her routine, for example, by a move to a retirement community. This may have caused enough stress to exacerbate the person's bipolar genetics.

◆ Due to vascular disease or other brain disease, the person may have organic brain damage which can look like bipolar disorder, though he or she does not carry the genes for it. In cases like this, lithium may not work, but valproate may. Lithium only seems to work with genetic bipolar disorder. Both of these drugs are significant in the management of bipolar disorder, but valproate works for seizures and organic damage, whereas lithium is used mainly for bipolar disorder.

Due to the episodic nature of bipolar disorder, it can appear at any time when there is an exacerbating environmental influence. In reality, the person has always had bipolar but it may not have developed into a disorder. He or she may not have shown obvious symptoms until something triggered an episode. The bipolar genetics would have been there first, except in the case of organic brain damage.

Triggers of Bipolar Disorder

It is important to distinguish between the genetic causes (underlying causes) and triggers (immediate perceptible causes and internal biological causes) of bipolar disorder. Hormones may trigger the bipolar disorder. Trauma may trigger the bipolar disorder. Poisoning the body with street drugs (another form of traumatizing the body) may trigger bipolar disorder. Traveling to a different time zone (usually over three hours' time change) or staying up all night may exacerbate bipolar disorder. Overwhelming stress may wake up the "bipolar monster" (as I sometimes call it). The triggers in this paragraph are the most significant triggers.

Previously we explained that the genes are the architects or planners, building and directing your body. The organs and structures like the thalamus and the adrenal gland are behaving and producing under their direction.

Your genes and organs are constantly reacting in response to external environmental stimuli. Environmental stressors are the triggers that turn on genes and the responses they provoke.

Hormones

It should be obvious that hormones have a significant effect on the bipolar genetics. Onset of bipolar symptoms usually happens in adolescence, when hormonal changes are emerging. Bipolar women will tell you that their bipolar disorder becomes the most symptomatic during a difficult premenstrual period.

Some women may go through life with no diagnosis (or even symptoms) of bipolar disorder until menopause, when chemical changes may aggravate a genetic predisposition toward bipolar disorder. What's the best way to treat this onset of bipolar disorder? Medication for bipolar disorder and treatment for the hormonal imbalance—in other words, treating her hormonal problem directly reduces her bipolar symptoms. Her hormonal imbalance may magnify her emotions, but then exacerbate her bipolar genetics, which multiplies the intensity of her emotions even more. A lot of empathy and understanding may be required from her loved ones during this time. And, by the way, don't take it personally.

Statistically, men are more prone to completing suicide than women. Typically men are prone to choosing methods of suicide that are more permanent, whereas women may choose less violent methods which can sometimes be reversed. Suicide, in bipolar disorder, is always a permanent solution for a temporary problem. However, among people with bipolar disorder, women commit suicide more often than men. Why? The type of hormonal problems that women have typically exacerbates bipolar disorder, as

Mental Note

Seasonal affective disorder (SAD) can trigger mood episodes, and some people with bipolar disorder become depressed during the sunless winter months. Needless to say, living in extremely cold climates where winter sunlight is diminished would not be advised for people with SAD and bipolar disorder.

mentioned in the last paragraph. The ratio of men to women with bipolar disorder is 50/50, so it is not a matter of more women having BP.

Trauma

As we have stated, trauma can trigger bipolar disorder. Some trauma cannot be avoided: loved ones get sick or die, people run red lights and crash into your car. When these things happen, a person with bipolar disorder needs to turn to his or her team of consultants.

Many soldiers who return from war exhibit bipolar symptoms that they'd never experienced prior to the traumatic experiences of combat. Likewise, people who survive a violent crime or other horrific experience may afterward exhibit bipolar symptoms for the first time. Often, these people are also suffering from post-traumatic stress disorder (PTSD). Combined with bipolar disorder, this makes for a very challenging mix, one that can take time to respond to treatment.

In these situations, the best course of action is usually to stabilize the patient with medication while also treating the PTSD. There are some good treatments available for post-traumatic stress now. EMDR (eye movement desensitization and reprocessing) can be beneficial in reducing or purging past trauma. Exposure therapy (a cognitive behavioral-therapy technique for reducing fear and anxiety) is also now supported by the Veterans Administration. Reducing the PTSD will also reduce the bipolar symptoms.

Sometimes an old trauma comes to life and looms over a person. A team of consultants is helpful during these times. Maybe the doctor needs to prescribe some adjunct medication during this time. Maybe it's time to visit the therapist, talk to a friend, and ask the family to have more patience. Ask someone to be your backup prefrontal lobe, in case yours falters. Have a team of "consultants" lined up: people that you trust when you are temporarily unable to operate at 100 percent. Try not to make any big decisions during these times. If you have to make a decision, call on a trusted loved one who seems to have your best interest at heart.

Illness or Injury

An illness or injury can exacerbate bipolar disorder. It may be time to call in your consultants to help you through. An illness or injury is essentially a trauma or a mini-trauma. And just as during a trauma, it would be in your best interest to have a backup person to help you navigate through this time.

Improper Drug Use

Recreational drug use is another common trigger of bipolar symptoms, stirring up the existing bipolar condition that may have gone undiagnosed until that point. On the other hand, sometimes people under the influence of drugs—especially amphetamines and other drugs that excite the system—may appear to be manic, when in fact they are not bipolar at all.

However, barring the known effects of a particular drug, a person who shows the whole range of bipolar symptoms is very likely to have bipolar disorder. To really know for sure, though, more investigation would need to be done. Does he have bipolar in his family? Can we eventually titrate him off the bipolar meds and see if he has another episode? Perhaps we should slowly take him off medication and watch him closely. This procedure is probably the right thing to do after only one episode.

Since people with bipolar disorder have the highest substance abuse of any mental health category, it is likely that they would need to be assessed for drug and alcohol rehab, detoxed from improper drugs, and given the right bipolar medication.

Stress

Job stress, marital stress, self-induced stress, and so on can all contribute to a person beginning to show symptoms of bipolar disorder. Looking for *pro-dromal indications* is helpful in avoiding a full-blown episode.

def•i•ni•tion

> **Pro-dromal indications** of a brewing bipolar episode include mood swings, fatigue, anger management problems, agitation, talkativeness, lack of insight, loss of big picture, lack of sleep, and so on. These may be not be severe enough to be diagnosable but may still be an indication of a bipolar cycle coming. The "bipolar monster" could be just over the horizon.

When a person has a tight deadline at work, this may create stress in his marriage, which in turn rebounds as more stress on the individual. If the individual is also driven to succeed excessively and has taken on too much responsibility, this can lead to an awakening of the bipolar monster. Two things are essential during these times:

- Having a person available who is familiar with the signs of an impending crash.
- Having a person to consult with confidentially (therapist, mentor, spiritual advisor).

A therapist who is familiar with bipolar disorder can be a saving grace. The therapist can work with the person who may have …

◆ Unrealistic goals or expectations.

◆ Perfectionism.

◆ Lack of insight, foresight, and hindsight.

◆ Lack of ability to relax, meditate, or have a realistic perspective.

◆ Anger management problems.

◆ Limited social skills.

◆ Limited interpersonal skills.

People who have bipolar disorder benefit greatly from developing relationship skills and interpersonal skills. These skills make life easier in the long run by reducing unnecessary stress.

Lack of Sleep

I believe that this is, by far, the biggest risk factor for exacerbating bipolar disorder. Lack of sleep can cause irritability, delusions, and even psychosis in any normal human being. It seems to be the biggest causal factor in exacerbating bipolar disorder. Students, for example, may stay up all night studying for an exam. People who do not have the genetics for BP may get away with this for a while, but people with BP genetics should never stay up all night. They should never work midnight shifts or swing shifts.

People with BP should try to establish a regimen of going to sleep at a decent hour and waking up at a decent hour. This is one of the biggest secrets to preventing symptoms of BP.

When I was on the staff at a local County Prison, a man came to JFK Airport from another country. The change in time zones had triggered a manic episode. This man was a wealthy businessman in his country,

 Red Flag

People who tend to have the genetics for bipolar disorder should never mess with their sleep. They should never stay up all night long. People with bipolar disorder also cannot work swing shift or third shift, and they must be very careful when visiting other time zones.

but one of his manic behaviors caused him to be arrested and brought to the prison. He hadn't slept from the mania, and from not having slept, he was delusional. He was in a country where no one looked like him, and he was paranoid from lack of sleep, so he wouldn't eat the food, sign any papers, or take any medication.

I was able to contact his sister, who flew in. He was able to take the medication when she was there approving. After that, he slept for a few days and was not psychotic. The best thing we could do for him was to allow him to fly back to his country in the custody of his sister.

Red Flag

People with BP must recognize and avoid the triggers that for them result in episodes. Some triggers are unavoidable, such as the death of a loved one, a divorce, and hormonal changes associated with the normal life cycle. Others are easier to avoid, such as drastic changes in sleep schedules due to work or play. Working the night shift or going out all night with friends can prove detrimental for someone with bipolar disorder.

That's an extreme example, but all of us have times when stress or circumstances disrupt our sleep schedules. People with BP would find relaxation techniques helpful for them get to sleep. In general, I don't believe people should take sleep medication, and I would counsel them in relaxation techniques. However, people with symptomatic bipolar disorder may need to take sleep medication. The alternative may be to have a manic episode that could ruin their lives or set them back. I have learned this lesson over years of treating people with bipolar disorder.

Bipolar is a blessing and a curse in many ways. The blessing is that you have to make sure you are in top condition, and you have to learn how to be interdependent with other people. A little humbleness and humility is always good for the soul. It helps curb the ego and the illusion that we don't need anyone else. In reality, we do need others. Better to realize that now, than wait until we are older and wiser. Developing interpersonal skills is one of the keys to success in life, no matter how it happens.

The Least You Need to Know

◆ Bipolar disorder is caused by genetic conditions, but other factors, like environmental conditions, can also play a role.

◆ Your bipolar disorder can remain "dormant" for a long time, until a contributing factor such as a major trauma triggers bipolar symptoms.

◆ Certain things are likely to trigger bipolar episodes. These include disrupted sleep patterns, major stress, or hormonal changes.

4

Diagnosis and Dual Diagnosis

In This Chapter

◆ An informal test for bipolar disorder

◆ Concerns about getting diagnosed

◆ The importance of dual diagnosis

You can't know for sure if you have bipolar disorder until you get an official diagnosis from a doctor. This is often a complicated process. The doctor may need to ask a lot of questions and perform some diagnostic tests (partly to rule out other conditions) before a definite diagnosis is possible. It would be a good idea if you asked the doctor to talk to a relative, spouse, or someone who knows you well and even ask if you can bring them in.

There is no physical test for bipolar disorder yet. Any diagnosis is based on the professional evaluation of the doctor or therapist or psychologist. In this chapter, we'll explain how a diagnosis is made and give you a basic test you can take yourself.

Could You Have Bipolar Disorder?

Bipolar disorder is a spectrum disorder, which means that even though you may not be diagnosable, you could still have some of the elements (features) of bipolar disorder. This test is based on the criteria given in the DSM-IV, which is published by the American Psychiatric Association, and also contains some new updated criteria based upon the International Conference on Bipolar Disorder (2007). It is not a formal test, but it should give you some idea if you may have bipolar disorder.

The best use of the test is to take it yourself and also have some relatives (or other people who know you well) take the test. Compare their answers to yours. If their answers are much different, that is a possible indication you could be bipolar. Keep in mind that most people show some of these elements at one time or another. Just answer the questions as honestly as you can.

A Self-Test

This is an informal bipolar test. It is not a professional diagnostic test. Mark your points for each question. Pick only ONE answer. If the answers don't fit, pick the closest one. If your answer is "no" or "none," put down zero for the points.

Have you ever had an inflated ego and felt that you were powerful (mentally or physically) for four days or more?

- ♦ If it "just happened" for no reason, give yourself 4 points.

- ♦ If you felt this way after accomplishing something big, give yourself 1 point.

- ♦ If it lasted for two days and you are under the age of 18, give yourself 2 points.

Points: ___

Have you had a decreased need for sleep lasting four days or more, where you felt rested after a few hours?

- ♦ If you didn't require any sleep for a couple days in a row, give yourself 4 points and skip the rest of this question.

- ♦ If you slept for three hours or less for four days and you felt rested, give yourself 3 points and skip the rest of this question.

- ♦ If you slept for six hours or less for four days and felt rested, give yourself 2 points and skip the rest of this question.

◆ If you didn't sleep much at night, but fell asleep during the day, give yourself 1 point.

◆ If you slept over 6 hours total out of 24 hours, give yourself 1 point.

Points: ___

Have you had four days or more where you were talkative and felt a pressure to keep talking?

◆ If you have had four days or more where you were much more talkative than usual and you couldn't stop talking, give yourself 4 points and skip the rest of this question.

◆ If you have had four days or more where you were much more talkative than usual, but you could force yourself to listen if you had to, give yourself 3 points and skip the rest of this question.

◆ If you are under the age of 18 and you have had two days where you couldn't stop talking, give yourself 2 points.

◆ If you were overly talkative after some big event in your life (good or bad) for a day or two, give yourself 1 point.

Points: ___

Have you had four days or more of racing thoughts, where your thoughts were coming faster than normal, or when you kept getting great ideas non-stop?

◆ If your thoughts during these days were so fast that you couldn't concentrate on any one thing for very long, give yourself 4 points.

◆ If you had a flight of ideas for four days or more or rapid thoughts for four days or more, give yourself 3 points.

◆ If you are under the age of 18 and you have had two days or more of racing thoughts, give yourself 2 points.

◆ If you have had a day or two that you couldn't stop thinking about a significant problem in your life, give yourself 1 point.

Points: ___

Have you had four days or more of elevated sexuality?

- ◆ If you have and you acted out sexually in a risky way (risk of pregnancy, risk of reputation, risk of getting a disease), give yourself 4 points.

- ◆ If you have and you did not act out and were able to control it, give yourself 2 points.

- ◆ If you have and you went against your own rules and then felt bad later, give yourself 1 point.

Points: ___

Have you experienced periods of excessive spending, binges of drug abuse, foolish investments, or sexual indiscretions?

- ◆ If you have done any of the above more than once, give yourself 3 points.

- ◆ If you have done any of these things once, give yourself 1 point.

Points: ___

Do people say you are moody? Do you have mood swings for no reason or very little reason?

- ◆ If this happens often, give yourself 3 points.

- ◆ If this happens because of events or hormonal changes, give yourself 1 point.

Points: ___

Do people say that you "say things without thinking"? Do people feel like you hurt their feelings when you are "honest"? Do you have difficulty imagining (or don't imagine) how the things you say are going to affect others?

- ◆ If any of the above is true, give yourself 3 points. If you are under the age of 18, give yourself 2 points.

- ◆ If you have times where you do this, but then feel badly afterward, give yourself 2 points.

- ◆ If you are mostly in control of what you say, give yourself 1 point.

Points: ___

Did you have temper tantrums lasting more than a half hour when you were a child?

- If so, give yourself 3 points.

- If not over a half hour, give yourself 1 point.

Points: ___

Do you get very upset anytime your plans have to change?

- If yes, give yourself 3 points.

- If only sometimes, give yourself 1 point.

Add up all your points: _____

If your total points are between 26 and 35, you need to be evaluated for bipolar disorder.

If you scored between 16 and 25, you would most likely benefit from an evaluation.

If you scored in the 5 to 15 range, you are within normal limits. If you scored a 3 or 4 on any one question, you may wish to talk with someone about that specific behavior, but it is unlikely that you have bipolar disorder.

If you scored 0 to 4, it is likely that you haven't answered the questions accurately.

What Do You Have to Lose?

The decision to visit a mental health professional is often difficult. It shouldn't be a source of shame or disappointment, but for many people it is. Centuries-old myths and misconceptions discourage even the most open-minded among us from seeking help.

You are not your heart or your liver; they are just your parts. You could be given someone else's organs and still be you, right? Your brain is special because it is "you." You can't get a brain transplant and still be you, right?

Wrong. It is theoretically possible to transfer the information in your brain to another—the technology may be coming (creepy, but very cool)! And even though your brain is different from your other organs, it is still susceptible to diseases and disorders. In the United States, one in five adults will suffer from a mental illness severe enough to cause them to seek treatment. So before we embark on our quest to lead happy and healthy lives, keep in mind that you are not alone.

In spite of these facts, many people who consider seeking psychiatric help are plagued by worries and embarrassment. We are here to tell you that you must do what is right for you, regardless of what anyone else thinks. An initial lack of acceptance is common, especially on the part of parents. Just remember to leave them a copy of this book and hope they read it. But even then it may take them a while to accept the "new" you. Most people who read up on this issue are easily persuaded to relax their fears and judgments. Don't ever allow the ignorance of others to stop you from having and enjoying the life you deserve.

In the realm of unawareness, many bipolar people are forced to get an evaluation by way of court order. Bipolar people who use illicit drugs and alcohol often have scrapes with the law. If you are arrested more than once for any of these things, chances are you will be sent to an addiction center for an evaluation and possibly treatment in addition to (or instead of) jail. A bipolar person may or may not be an addict, but many self-medicate with substances to an extent. The bottom line is, if a mental health professional had been treating a person with bipolar long before any arrest, the arrest probably would never have happened.

We believe being proactive will work to your benefit. It is better to act and fail than to fail to act. You may not find the right doctor or therapist or medication on your first attempt, but you will succeed if you are committed to your recovery.

Ways to Find Sources of Treatment

Once you've decided to seek treatment, you may be unsure how to go about getting it. Here are some smart moves in pursuit of dynamite treatment:

◆ Ask your friends if they have ever seen a psychiatrist or counselor. Many of them may have but won't mention it until you ask. If they haven't, they usually know someone who has. It gives you an opening to say you're thinking about it and possibly get their reaction.

◆ Ask your family doctor for a referral. Your doctor will usually have colleagues to recommend or a list of referrals he or she has heard great things about and trusts.

◆ If you are a college student, your school's health services often have great counselors and psychiatrists for free.

- If you are a veteran, the V.A. hospital will provide mental health services to you free of charge.

- If you are nervous about going for an evaluation, take a trusted friend with you to your appointment for moral support. Sometimes a close friend or family member can provide information that you have forgotten or do not know and help you get a proper diagnosis.

- Go to a publicly held group meeting specifically for bipolar people, like those held by the DBSA (Depression and Bipolar Support Alliance) or NAMI (National Alliance for Mental Illness). There is usually a NAMI chapter in every town and the meetings are free. You can sit and listen if you would rather not talk. People are known by their first names only and are there to share their experiences with doctors and medications. They can share coping skills that they have learned since recognizing their needs. Once you see that there are people from all walks of life, ages, and genders at the meeting, you may gather the courage you need to visit the psychiatrist and get a handle on your mood disorder. Who knows, you might even make some new friends!

Can I Afford It?

You don't have to be a Rockefeller to afford treatment. Many state, county, and community-based services are funded by charitable contributions. NAMI groups are free. The groups sponsored by the local mental health association are free. You may have some difficulty getting the right treatment, which is why it may benefit you to first go to these groups for ideas on treatment. They can best help you and tell you who has the best reputation.

 Mental Note _____

Hopefully it will be easy in your part of the country to locate free group meetings and public services on a "sliding scale" (fees based on your income or free). Using your Internet search engine and keywords like "bipolar" + the name of your city and state. Your local NAMI (National Alliance on Mental Illness) chapter or MHA (Mental Health Association) can guide you and can usually offer you group sessions at no cost.

"Employee assistance programs" are offered by many employers at little or no charge, providing access to mental health services, including individual or family counseling and treatment for substance abuse. Nearly every city has a local Mental Health Association with a listing in their phone book that will be glad to help you find appropriate services and groups. Drop-in services and appointment times are available day or night and on weekends and holidays, so no matter how hectic your work schedule, it is usually possible to find help.

Who Will Diagnose Me?

Many types of mental health professionals are available to you regardless of your income. You will have to do some research to find the right professional for you. We recommend that you describe your symptoms or problems to your family physician first. He or she can usually direct you to the type of mental health professional who will be most helpful.

- Psychiatrists: Medical doctors with special training in the diagnosis and treatment of mental illness, psychiatrists are able to prescribe medication and should have a state license and be certified by the American Board of Psychiatry and Neurology. Some psychiatrists specialize in diagnosing children with mental health problems.

- Psychologists: Psychologists who have completed a doctoral degree in psychology from an accredited program and have finished an internship of supervised professional experience are qualified to make evaluations and diagnoses and to provide individuals and groups with cognitive (talk) therapy. Some have private practices and others work for public organizations and hospitals.

- Clinical social worker: Counselors who have completed a Master's degree in social work from an accredited graduate program are qualified to render diagnoses and provide individual and group counseling. A clinical social worker should be licensed to work in your state and be a member of the Academy of Certified Social Workers.

- Licensed professional counselor: Counselors who have completed a Master's degree in psychology or counseling are qualified to diagnose mental disorders and provide individual and group counseling. They should be licensed to work in your state.

- Mental health counselor: Counselors who have completed a Master's degree in psychology or a related field and years of supervised clinical work are qualified to diagnose mental disorders and provide individual and group counseling. They should be certified by the National Academy of Certified Clinical Mental Health Counselors.

- Nurse psychotherapist: Registered nurses who are trained in psychiatric care and mental health nursing are qualified to diagnose mental disorders and provide individual and group counseling. A nurse psychotherapist has completed an accredited nursing program and medical certification and is state licensed.

- Marital and family therapist: Counselors who have completed a Master's degree in psychology or a related field and have specialized training in marital and family therapy are qualified to diagnose mental disorders and provide individual and group counseling. They should be licensed to work in your state.

- Nurse practitioners: They are able to prescribe medication and usually work under the guidance of a medical doctor. Some are trained in mental health and can usually give you more time than a medical doctor. In the case of a nurse practitioner, you get two professionals. The medical doctor supervises the nurse practitioner.

- Family doctor: Currently, fewer than 10 percent of family doctors are trained to treat bipolar disorder, but that number is changing. A therapist teamed with a family doctor who has training in bipolar disorder is the wave of the future. The therapist spends time with the patient and works with the doctor to get the right medication. The family doctor can usually see a patient in serious distress the same day or by the next day. If it a complicated case, the doctor can help with proper drugs until the patient can make an appointment with a psychiatrist.

Check that any of the preceding have been educated in bipolar disorder before making an appointment. It may even be her area of expertise. Ask a therapist or psychologist if she works with a particular doctor or nurse practitioner for bipolar disorder. If she doesn't work with any medical professionals, she may not have the expertise you need.

None of these professionals with different backgrounds and areas of expertise would exist—let alone be buried in patients—if no one was visiting them! Some psychiatrists haven't taken new patients in months or years due to the demand. As a result, psychiatrists customarily spend an hour with a patient the first visit but only 15 minutes with them at each subsequent session. They typically diagnose, prescribe, and then follow up during the short sessions to see if your medication has had the desired effects.

Psychotherapy or cognitive therapy is a very important part of a positive mental health outcome, and psychiatrists are now usually too busy to provide it. Choosing a counselor, psychologist, or social worker for individual therapy instead is very much in vogue—and usually cheaper.

How Will They Know?

Being diagnosed is the first step in formulating an effective treatment plan. The first step of diagnosis is to rule out any other physical or mental illnesses. In the future there may be a lab test for bipolar disorder, but that is many years away. Bipolar disorder must be diagnosed by a trained specialist. At present, diagnosticians use a manual called the DSM-IV to determine if you meet the criteria for bipolar disorder.

Mental health professionals will want to know everything. They may need information about your eating habits, sleeping patterns, energy level, emotional states, ability to concentrate, disturbed thoughts, and behavior. Often the first question they ask is, "What brings you here today?" The question may seem ridiculous at first, but it is typically an event-provoked breakdown that sends people to their first mental health visit. This could be a death, a divorce, a bad car accident, a firing, or something else. Unfortunately, most people don't go for help until they are amidst some disaster in their lives.

Mental Note

Before your appointment, think about and write down everything that you believe is relevant to why you are there. This includes symptoms, patterns, behaviors, diet routines, and so on. It's important to do this beforehand, because you may find yourself with mental block during your evaluation.

It is absolutely paramount to truthfully report all of your symptoms to the diagnostician and answer her questions as openly as possible. A survey showed that 28 percent of people with bipolar disorder held back some of their symptoms. It is pretty hard to help someone when the person is not honest. Confidentiality is protected. A psychologist, for example, can be sued and her license suspended for a breach in confidentiality. If she doesn't have a complete picture of your life, she will not be able to help you. Unprotected anonymous sex, illicit drug use, and screaming fits may be difficult for you to reveal during any first meeting. However, remember that the person you are telling has heard it all before and will not be surprised or judgmental in any way. Everything you divulge is strictly confidential and unless you grant permission for its release, it will stay that way.

If four or more of the symptoms listed in the DSM-IV have been present continually or most of the time for more than two weeks, chances are you will be diagnosed with bipolar disorder.

Dual Diagnosis

Over two-thirds of bipolar people have a concomitant or *comorbid* illness, meaning that they also suffer from another mental illness or a substance abuse problem in addition to the bipolar disorder. Fifty-seven to 60 percent of people with bipolar disorder do have a substance abuse problem. Many have secondary problems caused by their bipolar disorder, or by other factors.

Treating comorbid disorders is more complicated than treating either of the disorders alone. For one thing, certain medications commonly used to treat one condition may cause adverse affects in patients who also have the other condition (or can interact in a negative way with meds prescribed for that other condition). Sometimes you'll need to try a few different drug combinations to find the most effective therapy for you.

A program known as integrated dual diagnosis treatment is for people who are mentally ill and have an addiction. This treatment approach helps people recover by offering both mental health and substance abuse services at the same time and in one setting. The programs are not widely available, but it is worth your while to see if you are near a provider. They are long-term, community-based, comprehensive programs that have a good track record for preventing relapse among their participants.

def•i•ni•tion

Comorbidity means the presence of another disease or condition in a patient, in addition to the primary problem (in this case, bipolar disorder). The patient may seek treatment for both conditions simultaneously.

Mental Note

Mentally Ill Chemically Addicted (MICA) holds free support group meetings all over the United States. Your local mental health association can provide the times and dates if you have a local chapter.

Common Dual Diagnosis Conditions

Comorbid disorders most commonly diagnosed among bipolar patients are panic/anxiety disorders (including social phobia), obsessive compulsive disorder (OCD), post-traumatic stress disorder (PTSD), and impulse-control disorders like kleptomania and compulsive shopping. One of the most consistent things about bipolar disorder is that it is inconsistent. It may look like other things. The "anxiety" could be agitation from the bipolar disorder. If it is, the mood stabilizer will show a reduction in the "anxiety" in a few weeks. The "OCD" may be an obsessiveness that sometimes appears with agitated mania. Treatment of the mania reduces the "OCD" in this case. True OCD is always fear-driven. A person with OCD feels that something bad will happen if they don't perform certain rituals, like turning the lock in the door to check it five times.

Substance Abuse

Many people with BP have a substance abuse problem or a higher likelihood of developing one. Drug and alcohol experts tend to believe the addiction causes this behavior. Psychologists and medical people tend to believe that the bipolar disorder causes the tendency to self-medicate for the bipolar symptoms. It doesn't matter in that it's common for bipolar people to use drugs or alcohol. In either case, the treatment is the same, in that they should go a rehab to address the addiction issues, because when they are having bipolar symptoms, they are of an addict mentality and the rehab will help them deal with it.

Red Flag

Using drugs or alcohol while being treated for bipolar disorder is especially dangerous because many BP meds can have serious negative interactions with these other substances.

Whatever the root of the substance problem, it's important to treat it along with the bipolar disorder. Otherwise, it will be very difficult to see any improvement with either. If there is any addiction to the mania itself, this must also be treated as if it is a substance abuse problem.

Anxiety

Many people with BP think they suffer from anxiety, but this is often physical agitation linked to their BP. For people in this situation, a mood stabilizer can prove helpful. Bipolar sufferers probably will not find long-term relief from an anti-anxiety medication, which would normally be prescribed for anxiety in a person without bipolar disorder.

Attention Deficit Hyperactivity Disorder (ADHD)

Attention deficit hyperactivity disorder (ADHD) is often linked with bipolar disorder. Many BP patients are misdiagnosed with ADHD, while it is rare that BP patients may have ADHD as well as bipolar disorder. The problem is that symptoms exhibited during or after a manic phase can look similar to ADHD symptoms. After a manic episode, a six- to eight-week convalescence period is required before the brain's executive functions start functioning again. This can be mistaken for attention deficit.

Because the medications commonly prescribed to treat ADHD can trigger or heighten manic episodes, doctors usually proceed carefully when putting together a treatment plan for a BP patient who may also have ADHD. One psychiatrist at Hershey Medical Center first treats the mood and sleep problems, and then introduces ADHD meds after the person's bipolar disorder is stable. This seems to be the safest method.

Asperger's Syndrome

Also known as Asperger's disorder, this condition is part of the autism spectrum of disorders. Children with Asperger's syndrome are generally intelligent and function at a much higher level than those with other forms of autism. People with this condition often don't interact normally with other people. Among other things, they often avoid making eye contact.

While these same traits may sometimes be seen in a person with bipolar disorder (especially during a depressed episode), the difference is that a person with Asperger's will *always* display socially inept behaviors. A person with BP may only temporarily exhibit social miscues.

Obsessive Compulsive Disorder (OCD)

Obsessive compulsive disorder (OCD) is commonly diagnosed along with BP, but this diagnosis can be tricky because a lot of bipolar people do show "obsessive" traits that aren't caused by OCD. The medications for OCD usually interfere with treatment for BP, so the OCD should be verified completely before treatment is started. Some research shows that 10 to 12 percent of people with OCD have bipolar disorder. That is very high compared to the average of 1 to 3 percent of bipolar disorder in any population. Again, OCD behaviors are always fear driven. If it's not fear driven, it's not OCD.

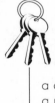

Mental Note _____

OCD habits are driven by fear. People with OCD perform certain rituals because of a fear that something bad will happen if they don't. People with BP, on the other hand, do things a certain way because that's how they want them, and doing things a different way irritates them. If you ask, "What would happen if you didn't do that?" a person with OCD would tell you that terrible things might occur. The person with BP might say, "I wouldn't like it."

Acceptance

Accepting your diagnosis may be tantamount to admitting to yourself that you are disabled to some degree. It's not easy for most bipolar people to do. Some of us believe we are better than other people in some ways, but at the same time suffer from deep-seated insecurities and even self-loathing. The truth is, bipolar sufferers may be more advanced than other people in certain ways—namely, we feel more. The best way to view your disorder is as a blessing and a curse. Successful treatment will minimize the role the disorder plays in your life.

People suffering from bipolar disorder are often reluctant to consider medication and therapy because their fear of losing themselves outweighs their fear of, well, themselves. Don't worry: the right medication and therapy will make you a better version of yourself. Most important, the medication(s) may liberate you from the control of your mood episodes.

Having been a victim of any cycle of abuse makes breaking that cycle difficult. Once you realize that you have been a victim of your mood episodes, you can stop making excuses for them and tell them they have to go! We promise you will not be brainwashed or explode when you start seeing a mental health professional or taking medication. You have nothing to lose and everything to gain.

Ultimately your prognosis (problem progression and chances for positive outcome) depends on many factors under your control: the right medicines, the right doses, a good working relationship with your treatment professional(s), a medical professional, a supportive and understanding therapist, and family, or a spouse. You also need to adopt a lifestyle that will regulate your stress levels, beginning with regular exercise and regular sleep and wake schedules.

The Least You Need to Know

◆ A short informal test may indicate the likelihood of bipolar disorder, but only a qualified professional can make a more definite diagnosis.

◆ Many different types of doctors and mental health professionals can diagnose BP if trained.

◆ Your doctor or mental health professional cannot effectively help you unless you are totally honest and forthcoming with him or her.

◆ It's important to keep a positive outlook. While getting an official diagnosis can be scary, it's the first step toward managing your symptoms and taking control of your life.

◆ The majority of people with bipolar disorder also suffer from a substance abuse problem or another mental health problem.

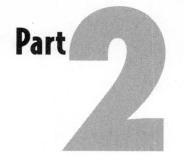

Part 2

Symptoms/Effects of Bipolar Disorder

In this part, we'll look at the symptoms caused by bipolar disorder—from the major ones like mania and depression to less severe (yet still annoying) ones like weight gain. We'll also discuss what to do when symptoms reach a critical point and talk about the special issues faced by young people with bipolar disorder.

Chapter 5

Manic Phases

In This Chapter

- Manic behavior perceptions and misperceptions
- The cause of mania
- How to cope with manic behavior

If bipolar disorder is a series of ups and downs, then mania is the "up" part of the equation. On the surface, that might seem good—hey, everybody likes being "up," right? However, the manic part of BP can cause just as many problems as the depression part. Mania shows up as euphoria, anger (which is actually internal rage), or anxiety (which is actually agitation). In this chapter, we'll explain what mania is, what causes it, and how you can cope with it.

Causes and Triggers of Mania

A recent study by the National Institute of Mental Health (NIMH) showed that a person's risk of developing bipolar disorder is influenced by a variation in a gene called DGKH. The gene manufactures a PKC (protein kinase C)–regulating protein that can be found in standard medications for bipolar disorder.

Gamma-aminobutyric acid (GABA) is a neurotransmitter that inhibits other neurotransmitters. It acts as a thermostat, regulating brain chemicals such as dopamine, norepinephrine, and serotonin. It is believed that low levels of GABA are associated with mania. With GABA levels below average, the brain is excessively stimulated.

You might think that drinking a glass of GABA could cause your mania to cease. It doesn't work that directly. If I broke my leg on a Friday, I can't take a bunch of calcium and magnesium and have it heal by Monday. All I would get was gas. It is a body process that has its own time table. There are other things going on in the brain. We actually don't know a lot about the brain and the mechanisms by which neurotransmitters work. Nobody looks in a microscope and says, "Ooh, look! There's that GABA thing stopping that dopamine thing from exciting the dopamine center!"

Triggers don't cause mania by themselves (although it may look that way). Mania is caused by a genetic condition and is set off by something (stress, excessive thinking, infatuation, trauma, and so on), causing chemical changes in the brain. Let's leave the brain chemical causes to the medical field and concentrate on the triggers, which we can control.

Triggers vary with the individual. Lack of sleep can trigger a manic episode, as well as any change in circadian rhythm (sleep patterns), such as traveling across several time zones. It is now well known that certain antidepressant medications (tricyclics and SSRIs) can trigger a manic episode. Some manic episodes are triggered by excessive anger (adrenaline).

Some people say that thinking too much can trigger an episode for them. They have trouble in college because they are thinking, thinking, thinking all the time, which triggers racing thoughts, which triggers mania. Sexual attraction triggers mania for some people. Being "in love" can trigger it for some. Some people with bipolar disorder actually learn to avoid people they are attracted to because it triggers their mania. These triggers have common threads with the elements of mania:

- Racing thoughts
- Hypersexuality
- Anger (rage)
- Euphoria

The trick is to find out what triggers manic episodes for you and to learn to avoid, defuse, or better manage those situations. A good cognitive behavioral therapist who is familiar with BP can help discover and list your triggers. Your therapist will likely ask you, "What precipitated your last episode?"

Sometimes PTSD (post-traumatic stress disorder) can trigger a manic episode. Imagine a man who had a rough childhood. His father would get drunk at Christmas and physically abuse his wife and children. This traumatized the man when he was a child. He never drank, but when Christmas rolled around, he would become agitated. The closer to Christmas day it became, the more sleep he lost and the more agitated he became. Almost every year, he had a manic episode around Christmas and needed to be admitted to the hospital. This is a typical example of mania triggered by PTSD.

Signs and Symptoms

Kristin Finn, author of *Bipolar and Pregnant*, wrote a great description that illustrates the signs and symptoms of mania. She had gone off her medication to accommodate her pregnancy and the sidebar contains her journal entry (reprinted by permission of HCI Books, Inc.).

Of course, the biggest problem with mania is that you lose the ability to see yourself. In a few cases, people have been filmed during a manic episode. Later, when they were shown the film, they couldn't believe how they were acting. A person has no perspective when manic. Many times he or she doesn't remember himself or herself that way during that time.

You lose the ability (in whole or part) to put yourself in another's place. Someone might think you are being rude or callous. Maybe you didn't mean to be rude or callous. You may think the person is "too sensitive," but take a look at your actions. If you can't seem to be introspective about your actions, and if you assess them with thought only, you may be a little manic. If you are very manic, you may not be able to see any of the signs.

I have never heard of anyone saying, "I feel a little manic right now, so I hurt your feelings because I can't really put myself in your place or imagine how you feel." If someone could say that, they would have insight. But you don't get insight with mania. You only get thoughts. Maybe they are brilliant thoughts, but they are just thoughts.

It is a good idea to have a trusted friend, spouse, or relative observe your actions during a manic episode. The bond that you have with others can override the ego, arrogance, entitlement, and lack of insight. No one can say a person who is manic is "thoughtless." The person has plenty of thoughts—don't argue with him or her about that. The person just may not be able to see the context behind the term "thoughtless," which actually translates into "insightless," "unempathetic," or "foresightless."

> ### Real People
>
> Following a documented action plan and my previous journal entries helped me to focus on our goal of having a second baby. Again, ongoing communication with my psychiatrist was an important part of the process. Even though I anticipated experiencing temporary manic and depressive episodes, at [the] time they seemed so permanent.
>
> In this next journal entry I describe a manic episode.
>
> *January 14, 1994, A.M.:* My mind is racing so fast I don't know where to begin. I feel as if I'm on a train (on the outside hanging on, not in a comfortable seat inside) going really fast. I wish I could jump off to slow myself down.
>
> *When I'm having a conversation with someone, it's hard for me to follow them at their slow pace. My mind processes the information at such a fast rate. I feel as if I know where their conversation is going before they verbalize it to me.*
>
> *I know this will pass. I have a feeling I'll see improvement (experience peace of mind again) once I get pregnant. Once I'm pregnant I will be able to see the light at the end of the tunnel (I'll be closer to being able to go back on lithium).*
>
> *Two minutes later—I felt so isolated. Not many people understand what I'm going through. I just caught myself going through my phone book looking for someone I could call to talk with—someone who can identify with how I'm feeling.*
>
> I vividly remember this experience. I felt so desperate and hopeless. I ended up not calling anyone to share how I was feeling. I truly thought no one could understand or relate to my racing mind or my feelings of isolation.
>
> *January 14, P.M.:* I feel a lot better now. Fred just got home and I'm looking forward to a nice, quiet weekend with him and Katherine.
>
> As you can see, there were days when I felt as if I were on an emotional roller coaster. These January 14 excerpts are an excellent example of temporary bipolar phases. I referred to them when I needed to be reminded that these agonizing feelings were not permanent. It helped me to keep things in perspective.

Memory Troubles

Another sign of a manic episode is effects on the memory. This is important. Mania comes with a lack of perspective. Without seeing context, you can't have perspective. You may not remember things the way others remember them. This concept is so important to understanding mania that we will give three examples of memory problems that manic people don't realize they have.

Confabulation

You will find confabulation in an intelligent drunk. You ask him how he got to your house, and he can't remember because he was drunk. He is embarrassed by this, so he thinks, *Well, I couldn't have driven my car because I smashed it up the other night, and I couldn't have taken a taxi because I have no money.* So he tells you, "I walked."

Later you find out that Joe drove him. You confront him, asking, "Why did you lie to me? Joe drove you in."

He responds, "Oh, yeah, that's right. Joe drove me in."

You could spend the rest of the day trying to figure out why he lied to you. Maybe he is a pathological liar. Maybe he didn't want you to know that Joe picked him up for some reason. But why would he do that? He was confabulating.

People with bipolar disorder may have memory blanks when manic. Manic episodes can have results similar to those of taking amphetamines, and amphetamines are known to have effects on memory. Those who take them may not remember conversations they had or certain events of the day.

Brain Chemical Surge

A 10-year-old diagnosed with BP comes down in the morning for breakfast, and Mom gives him his cereal and his meds. During breakfast, he gets angry and calls his mother a bad word. She sends him upstairs, saying, "Go to your room and don't come down until you have a different attitude."

He stomps up to his room and comes back down 10 minutes later. He hugs his mom and tells her he loves her. She says, "Well, that's a lot better than calling me a bad word!"

He looks at her funny and says, "I didn't call you a bad word!"

She says, "You certainly did. You father heard you say it."

The father agrees. The kid backs off because he has been through this before. What happened?

Children with bipolar disorder are rapid cyclers and may have ups and downs a couple times a day. This kid's brain chemicals peaked this morning. How do we know this child is not a liar? Because he wasn't dumb enough to think he could say that in front of his father and his mother and get away with it. A poll of my seminar attendees revealed that this type of behavior is common among bipolar children.

Psychogenic Amnesia

Psychogenic amnesia is another possible symptom of mania. A 50-year-old woman worked for a church. BP ran in her family, but she had never had symptoms herself. She had been taken in by her grandparents when she was 3, and they provided a stable life for her. She had gone to Bible college, where she met her beloved husband, and they had a wonderful marriage.

def•i•ni•tion

Psychogenic amnesia is a psychological amnesia that is caused by severe denial.

The minister asked this woman to show a prospective new member the church on the Friday of a week he would be at a convention. Her father died suddenly on Monday of that week. On Wednesday, her husband had a heart attack, and it didn't look like he was going to make it. She hardly slept. On Thursday, the woman was wandering around the church and had a full-blown manic episode. She became hypersexual and had an encounter with the janitor in the rectory. Later that day, her doctor gave her a sleeping aid and she slept through the afternoon and all night long. On Friday, she was showing the prospective member through the church and the janitor saw her. He asked, "Are you okay? Are you sure you're all right?"

She became nervous and wondered why the janitor would ask that. She had completely blocked the memory of the encounter with him. Psychogenic amnesia had blocked memories that she couldn't confront: that she loved her husband, but had relations with another man.

When the minister returned, she told him that the janitor was behaving strangely. The minister asked the janitor about it and the janitor spilled the beans about the encounter in the rectory. The minister didn't believe him and fired him on the spot.

Over the next month, the woman started having flashbacks (as can happen with psychogenic amnesia). After a time she realized what she had done. Being a righteous woman, she confessed it to the minister.

Common Traits

The common traits of mania are …

- ◆ Grandiosity and ego. The DSM-IV calls it "inflated esteem." It's not esteem, it's ego. Esteem comes from nurturing and a general confidence about oneself. Ego is self-centered, while esteem includes others.

◆ Decreased ability to sleep. The person feels as if he has no need to sleep (though he does, of course, as the crash at the end of the episode will show).

◆ Being talkative and unable to stop. Some say the brain is "directly connected to the tongue." If the person does stop talking, you can tell she is not really listening to you. She is just waiting until she can talk.

◆ Racing thoughts. So many ideas! The person feels as if his thoughts are moving along the mental highway at 100 miles per hour.

◆ Being distracted; dwelling on unimportant details and missing or not being interested in the bigger picture.

◆ Being goal-directed at school, socially, sexually, and otherwise.

◆ Agitation (which may be perceived as anxiety).

◆ Being unable to assess the risk or see the consequences in pleasurable activities (spending, sex, drugs, get-rich-quick schemes).

◆ Arrogance and entitlement (to go along with ego above). Not everyone who shows these traits has bipolar disorder, of course. With bipolar disorder, these traits are temporary. For others, they may be an aspect of their personality. It is likely to not be about personality for someone with BP.

◆ Mood swings. For example, a person may switch easily from euphoric mania to rageful mania.

A person may officially be having a manic episode if three of the preceding traits (which are abnormal for that person) last more than a week.

Manic Hyper Behavior

A person who appears to be hyper and manic is most likely agitated. That agitation can feel like anxiety, which people deal with in various ways. Some people become overactive; some feel panic and freeze. Others become aggressive. Some newer research links the adrenal gland to mania, but the results aren't in yet.

Ninety-three percent of bipolar kids show symptoms that could be diagnosed as attention deficit hyperactivity disorder, but they are not ADHD. If they get diagnosed as ADHD, someone will probably put them on a psychostimulant, which is like putting the child on rocket fuel, and that should be avoided.

Rage

Bipolar disorder can trigger never-ending rage. This manic "anger" is not true anger. True anger can have a *catharsis* (release), a purging of emotion. (The word comes from a Greek word meaning "purify.") If you have a good cry after true anger, you may feel better. If you are able to express your anger, you may feel better.

So if someone walks up to you and starts yelling at you, you may think to yourself, "I'll just let them yell at me for a while and get it out of their system. Then we'll talk."

That's usually a good idea, if you are up to it, but not with bipolar rage. The anger you see in mania is not anger. It is rage. Rage does not lead to catharsis, because rage begets rage. An enraged person will yell at you from now until next Tuesday and only get more and more enraged. The best way to deal with a person like this is to "switch him." You may try to redirect his anger toward someone who is not present or you may ask, "What are you so sad about?" (Many times manic anger is actually sadness.) There are a variety of different "switches"; just don't let an enraged person go on and on. Rage is likely to get worse and worse until something "switches" it to euphoria or "anxiety." This author's favorite switching tool is to use humor.

> **Real People**
>
> A man with bipolar disorder became enraged while drinking in a bar in Boston. He called his estranged wife in another state to come and get him. She refused. Though she had a restraining order against him, he said he was coming home. When she asked him how he was going to get there, he said, "I'll walk." Because he was manic and goal-directed, he walked from Boston to his home in another state, walking through the night. It took days for him to get home, and the police greeted him at his door, where he was whisked off to jail, diagnosed with BP, and finally treated.

Impulsive Behavior

Without the prefrontal lobe working and no insight, foresight, or hindsight, a person is liable to be very impulsive, with no ability to see the consequences of his or her actions.

Once I worked with an inmate who was threatening to punch out his corrections officer (CO). The inmate (who I suspected had bipolar disorder) was normally a nice guy, so the treatment specialist asked me to talk to him.

The inmate was only two weeks from his release. He told me he was going to punch out the CO (acting as if his brain were directly connected to his tongue). He said the CO had disrespected him by calling him a knucklehead. I asked him if he wanted to be home with his family. He said yes. I said, "If you punch out the CO, you won't be able to go home."

It was like an insight for him. He was a smart guy, but he hadn't visited his prefrontal lobe lately. He asked what he should do. I told him that if I were him, I would say, "Thank you," to whatever the CO said and be out in two weeks. He took me literally. In the cafeteria, the CO came over and asked me, "What did you tell that guy? Everything I say to him, he says, 'Thank you.' I think you are making these people nuts, Carter."

Actually, this particular man would not go on medication because he insisted he "wasn't nuts." I hope he has found a substitute prefrontal lobe to guide him (maybe his parole officer), because it didn't look like he was going to fire up his own with medication anytime soon. He wasn't really a criminal; he was in jail for self-medicating with illegal drugs. Luckily we stopped him before he had a chance to throw a punch at his CO.

Arrogance

Usually arrogance is a mask for a lack of confidence. People who lack confidence may display arrogance as a way of compensating for the way they feel. I remember when I was in high school, walking into school like I owned it, with a sway and a mean look on my face, secretly hoping no one would see through my act and kick my butt.

You often see arrogance in mania. It is part of the trilogy of ego, arrogance, and entitlement. Arrogance may look like confidence, but it isn't with mania. It is chemically induced. If you took amphetamines, you might start thinking faster and feel mentally "sharp." Your feelings of superiority might surface as you rose above the rest of us mortals, and you might act and feel confident as you made an ass out of yourself. The same reaction occurs in mania.

Addiction to the Mania

Some people with BP are unable to see the downside of mania. They actually become addicted to it. Imagine waking up one morning feeling really good. Your pupils look funny because the dopamine centers in your brain are unbalanced. You are thinking faster than other people. Your ego is through the roof. You are arrogant, but it feels like confidence. You have a sense of entitlement. You sail through the day brilliantly. You are not afraid to talk to people because you have important things to convey. One of your friends sees the way you are acting, looks at your pupils, and says, "What are you on?"

You reply enthusiastically, "I'm not on anything. Just high on life. That's all! Just high on life!"

Eventually, your loved ones become concerned about you and take you to see a doctor. You hear the doctor say, "Hey, you feel a little bit too good. We need to give you some medication to make you feel less good, so you can join us down here on Earth, okay?"

Are you going to go for that? Probably not!

Real People

A brilliant woman with multiple academic degrees and working for a prestigious organization had a manic episode in a large city. She had never felt better in her life. She had a great "insight" about possessions, "knowing" she didn't need them. She gave away her credit cards and the clothes on her back. Someone called the psych ward and they came and picked her up. She didn't sleep. Eventually she became psychotic, thinking the FBI was after her and that there were listening devices in the wall. The paranoia and angst created a horrible experience she would never want to repeat.

The woman was very compliant with her medication after the episode. She wasn't prone to addiction, so she didn't try to reduce her meds to get "that energy" or do any of the things that addicts do to deceive themselves. She wasn't going to do anything to create that mania again. But she has said that she remembers how good she felt when the mania first took her. She said that she would love to feel that way again—but without the consequences.

This type of euphoric mania is difficult to treat because people don't want to give it up. Addiction is not about drugs or alcohol. It's about the mentality underneath the drugs or alcohol. It's about looking for anything that gets a person high or relieves him or her from experiencing negative feelings.

A woman at a rehab facility where I worked went off her lithium. Mania is likely to occur when someone goes off lithium suddenly. I called her into my office with my "Tough Love" poster to ask her why she went off her lithium. She said, "Because I'm not personable on my lithium."

I have heard all the addict talk, like, "I'm not quick on my feet when I'm on my medication," "I am not creative on my meds," or "I have more energy off my meds."

I said, "I see. You went off your medication to get high."

She responded, "I am not using drugs!"

I was more emphatic when I said, "You don't have to buy drugs to get high. All you have to do is go off your lithium. What have you done to deserve being personable? Have you taken any communication classes or interpersonal communications in college?"

"Well, no," she said.

"Then you don't deserve to be personable. You haven't earned it. You are cheating, just like the guy who has to have a few drinks before he goes to a party to loosen up. Instead of learning how to be more personable, he cheats. You might think you are more personable when you are manic, but other people don't share that opinion. You need to go back on your lithium. Maybe you could take a Dale Carnegie course to become more personable. That way, you will have developed your ability to be personable instead of cheating by going off your meds."

To her credit, she went back on her lithium.

Human beings can be addicted to anything. It isn't always drugs or alcohol. It could be work, food, sex, or chocolate. If there was a chocolate rehab, I'd have to think about admitting myself.

Like any addiction, a person loses track of the bigger picture. This is magnified when the person has symptoms of bipolar disorder, because one of the symptoms of mania is a blackout of the bigger picture—the consequences.

SPECT scans have shown that the prefrontal lobe doesn't resume working normally for about 100 days after a cocaine addiction ends. There is very little activity in the lobe for six to eight weeks, meaning the person is unable to have foresight, insight, or hindsight. After six to eight weeks the lobe returns, but doesn't function at 100 percent until about 100 days.

The timeline for mania is not much different, so don't play with your meds to get "that energy." If you decide to go for the mania, misery is around the next corner. Some say that the prefrontal lobe is the seat of the soul. If so, you are literally trading your soul to get high.

Post-Manic Recovery

After a manic episode, a person has no prefrontal lobe (insight). He may not be able to focus (see the big picture, context, or themes). He is probably fatigued from lack of sleep, overactivity, and racing thoughts. The serotonin level in his brain is likely to be low. The person will probably sink into a depression, if he hasn't already. He may have done things to ruin his relationships, job, and financial security, and his actions may have legal consequences.

When the lobe starts coming back (six to eight weeks later) and the person sees the harm he may have done to his loved ones, career, reputation, and so on, he may become suicidal. He may think his loved ones would be better off without him. He may have had another episode and be tired of starting over, again and again.

The person needs to be assured that his brain will start working in six to eight weeks. He needs assurance that the meaning in his life will become more apparent once he has the part of the brain that can see the meaning in life back. At this low point, after he may have caused so much grief, is when he will need support the most. He will need help and assurance in taking his meds. He cannot be trusted to take them consistently with his brain temporarily malfunctioning.

The person may seem petty or superficial because he truly doesn't see the bigger picture. Don't take it personally. Don't think that this is who he is. It's not. Again, bipolar disorder is not a personality problem. It is not an ethics problem.

Some people have been diagnosed with depression with underlying anxiety or anxiety with underlying depression. Sometimes these people have been through all the standard antidepressants (SSRIs and tricyclics) to no avail. It is possible that bipolar medication (that has an antidepressant quality) will work for them. Do they have bipolar disorder? Who knows? But we do know that there are other disorders we haven't defined yet in the DSM. Is their anxiety actually an underlying suppressed mania? Who knows?

The main point is that bipolar medication like lithium, quetiapine, or lamotrigine may slowly dissipate their anxiety and depression.

The Least You Need to Know

- Mania can appear in the form of euphoria, anger, or anxiety.
- Some people with bipolar disorder are unable to see the negative effects of their manic episodes and are therefore reluctant to try to stop them.
- It can take several weeks for someone to recover from a manic episode and realize the effects of his or her actions.

Chapter 6

Bipolar, Depression, and Suicide

In This Chapter

- ◆ Is it depression or fatigue?
- ◆ The heightened risk of suicide
- ◆ The role of the prefrontal lobe
- ◆ Regrets and guilt from manic behavior

Bipolar disorder is also known as manic-depression, because it involves mania and depression. We discussed one half of the equation (mania) in the previous chapter. In this chapter, we'll talk about the depression associated with bipolar disorder.

Bipolar Depression

As we said in the last chapter, after a manic episode and the subsequent crash, the prefrontal lobe is off-line for six to eight weeks. During this period, the person usually experiences a depression that can range from moderate to severe. In this depressed state, the person may not be able to see the meaning in life, let alone take pleasure in it. She may not be able to focus, because the ability to see the big picture or the context of anything has taken a hiatus for a couple months.

The good news is, it will come back. You will get your brain back. You will be able to see the meaning in your life. There is hope for the future, even if you can't see it, and even though it doesn't seem that way or feel that way. Depression is a temporary state that feels like it has been there forever and will be there forever. During this time, don't make permanent decisions to solve temporary problems. Whatever messes you made during your mania will not seem so insurmountable once you get your prefrontal lobe back.

Mental Note _____

Johns Hopkins University Medical Center found that after a manic episode, there is up to 40 percent less serotonin in the brain. Lack of serotonin in the brain is associated with hostility and depression.

Depending on how much sleep you lost and how fast your mind was spinning during your manic episode, you may have chronic fatigue afterward. Chronic fatigue looks just like depression—the difference is in the motivation (or lack thereof). With chronic fatigue, you have the desire to do things, but you feel physically unable to. With depression, you have no desire or motivation at all. You may be depressed and/or chronically fatigued for a couple months after a manic episode.

Understanding Bipolar-Related Depression

You should know some things about depression. First of all, depression is the body's way of recuperating after certain events. After a trauma, for example, most people go into shock, which can look like depression.

Some people believe that depression is the body and mind's way of going off-line to heal from both physical and mental traumas. Some mental health professionals believe that it is a natural and necessary part of the healing process.

A true physical depression that isn't a bipolar depression and isn't the result of mania is usually treatable with the standard SSRIs, tricyclics, or an SNRI (serotonin norepinephrine reuptake inhibitor). Some physical depression runs in families and may involve a lack of serotonin or norepinephrine. For example, venlafaxine is an SNRI that increases both serotonin and norepinephrine. After taking this medication, a person may say, "I feel like myself again."

The same medications may not work for people with bipolar disorder. They may feel "too good" on this medication, which means the medication has stimulated the mania, or they may have a full-blown manic episode. If it is used, the newest research shows that these medications (SSRI, tricyclics) have no efficacy for bipolar depression.

If mania has caused someone to be overactive and not sleep, it may be too much to expect that an antidepressant will help. The person needs rest and his or her brain may need to recuperate. A psychostimulant would just sap more energy from the body. What goes up ...!

Bipolar depression can be very difficult to treat. Only a few medications work well and quickly for some people with BP. Other meds will work, but may take some time. It may be difficult for someone with BP to know if the meds prescribed are improving his or her health. If you are depressed and someone asks how your meds are working, your first impulse is to say, "They're not." But if the doctor asks you to remember how you felt when you came in a month ago and asks if you feel better now, you may see the improvement. Regardless, it is a gradual recovery process.

Symptoms of Bipolar Depression

The signs and symptoms of the depressive phase of bipolar disorder include unrelenting sadness. It may seem like everything is lousy, always was lousy, and always will be lousy. It may seem that any happiness you enjoyed was phony and fleeting. The hopelessness pervades your body and thoughts like a virus. You may not be able to function at all, and if you are, you feel like a robot going through the motions. You may think that you don't matter and that everyone would be better off without you—no matter what anyone tells you. You may take no pleasure in anything that gave you pleasure before. It may seem like there is nothing you can do about this. You may feel powerless, insignificant, and just a shell of your former self. It seems like this will go on forever.

The good news is that "forever," in the case of a depression following a manic episode, may last only six to eight weeks. The bad news is that those weeks feel like forever, no matter what anyone says. You wouldn't be surprised if someone said to you, "Due to the energy crisis, we have shut off the light at the end of the tunnel."

Common symptoms of depression include ...

♦ Deep feelings of hopelessness, loneliness, helplessness, and worthlessness

♦ Confusion and difficulty concentrating

♦ Self-loathing

- ◆ Apathy or indifference
- ◆ Loss of libido
- ◆ Withdrawing from social aspects and people
- ◆ Lethargy
- ◆ Morbid obsessions (romanticizing suicide and death)

Mental Note _____

Most people find this surprising, but anger can be a common symptom of depression. Anger is one step above apathy and can be an indication of someone trying to fight apathy. Apathy can also be the lid on a barrel of anger, suppressing real anger. In the movie *Anger Management,* Adam Sandler's problem was that he *never* got angry. Anger is a part of everyday life. To the degree you suppress one feeling, you suppress them all. Many people coming out of a depression find themselves becoming angry. It can actually be a sign of improvement. You just have to make sure you direct your anger so you don't make your life more difficult.

There are plenty of ways to relieve anger. Running, other forms of exercise, and writing are acceptable ways to relieve yourself of anger. One of the best maintenance tactics for people with BP seems to be vigorous exercise. You have to be careful not to let anger turn into rage and trigger mania.

The symptoms must last for two weeks and make it difficult for the person to function in order to meet the criteria for a depressive episode.

Research Says

The vast majority of people diagnosed with bipolar disorder suffer from depression more often than any other type of symptom.

In some particularly serious cases, an individual may experience psychosis while he or she is depressed, a condition also known as "severe bipolar depression with psychotic features." Many times it is a lack of sleep that is at cause, but it could also be a severe chemical imbalance.

Suicide

One of the causes of the high suicide rate with bipolar disorder is that bipolar disorder is a square peg that doesn't fit in the round holes of our mental health laws. You have to be an immediate danger to yourself or others before you can be committed against your will. That does not work for people with bipolar disorder. Most of our states have laws forbidding the mandatory admission of someone to the psych ward unless they are an immediate danger.

At this writing, only one state makes an exception to this. That is why the suicide rate for people with bipolar disorder is over 19 percent. We believe that it is actually higher than that because there are people who are undiagnosed with bipolar disorder who commit suicide. That would bring it up to approximately 25 percent. That is one out of four people. Usually they do it within the first two years after onset; if they don't do it then, they will probably not do it.

Unfortunately, we allow people who are manic to ruin their lives before we help. One such person said, "Oh, so now that I have ruined my life, gambled away my life savings, ruined my marriage, and lost my job, you want to save me because I threatened to commit suicide? Where were you before I did all the damage? Yes, I refused treatment, but I was crazy!"

Clearly we need to allow people with bipolar disorder to sign up and be an exception to that rule. When a person with bipolar disorder is lucid, they are very likely to say, "Hey look, I am bipolar. If I start acting manic and doing crazy things, you can admit me against my will, and I won't sue." There may be a way to get help by appointing a mental health power of attorney ahead of time as described next.

If you have bipolar disorder and you have refused treatment when you needed it (or fear that you may do so at some point), you can make up a mental health power of attorney and assign someone else to make the decision of admission. Your power of attorney document must say that you won't sue the facility, and it must be "irrevocable" and have a time limit on it. In many states, the power of attorney must go to a psychiatrist or psychologist with admitting privileges.

 Mental Note _____

One state will allow a person on an exception list to be committed. If a person promises not to sue, he can be admitted against his will during an episode. The only political hurdle is to get managed care to pay for the admission. When all states adopt this concept, the suicide rate for bipolar disorder will come down significantly.

Example I: If parents have a son who is approaching legal age, but he has not demonstrated that he can manage his bipolar disorder, he can sign a mental health power of attorney, extending his parents' rights (or assigning a psychiatrist the right) to admit him against his will until a later age.

Example II: If a bipolar woman wants to get pregnant, she can sign a mental health power of attorney to protect herself when she goes off her medication to get pregnant. The time period may be made to cover her from the moment she goes off her medication to about six months after she has the baby.

Red Flag

People with bipolar disorder commit suicide at a rate 14 times greater than normal. People who are bipolar with anxiety have a 36 times greater chance of committing suicide. People who are bipolar without anxiety have only a 7 times greater chance.

Another major cause of suicide, within the bipolar symptoms, is the extraordinary agitation that can be overwhelming and all consuming. People experiencing this high agitation may say, "I can't stand to be in my own skin. I want to die right now, rather than feel this way for another second." Those kind of comments indicate how consuming it can be.

Statistics show that people who are bipolar with "anxiety" have the highest rate of suicide, but that doesn't make phenomenological sense. Most likely, physical agitation is being mistaken for anxiety in these cases. Agitation may feel exactly like anxiety, but the causal source is different. Much anxiety can be treated psychologically, whereas the source of agitation is usually a physical source. Benzodiazepines (the drugs usually prescribed when a person says they have anxiety) merely mask the symptoms of agitation, whereas a mood stabilizer is likely to take care of the source of the agitation.

The bipolar sufferer at the greatest risk of suicide is likely to be a woman in her first two years of onset, with agitation (perhaps mislabeled "anxiety"). This is why it is of paramount importance to distinguish between the two. Agitation and anxiety cannot usually be distinguished by the way they "feel," so the source of the "feeling" must be established. Is the person bipolar? If so, it is most likely agitation. Does this person have hypervigilence (shaking of the foot, tapping, and so on)? Those are signs of agitation even if the person says, "I feel anxiety." Most people cannot perceive the difference and do not think of the word "agitation" unless educated on the meaning of that word.

It would not make sense to treat a bipolar person with agitation, with an antipsychotic alone, as antipsychotics can actually cause agitation in some people. Since the suicide rate is so high among people with agitation, a true mood stabilizer might be a better medication. If you see a doctor treating agitation with an antipsychotic alone, ask about it. The doctor may be treating the agitation as anxiety with antianxiety medication because the patient complains of "anxiety."

What Should I Do If I'm Depressed?

If you begin to feel depressed, the first thing you must do is see a doctor and make him or her aware of the problem. Don't wait until you are paralyzed by depression to seek preventative care. If you have experienced past bouts of depression, you may almost certainly have more—and perhaps worse—bouts in the future. Research has shown that mood episodes increase in severity over time. Don't make the mistake of thinking bipolar depression will resolve itself without intervention. The odds are it won't. The thing you have going for you is that you have dealt with it before and can sharpen your coping skills to avoid it or deal with it better than before.

Of course, the best way to treat depression is to avoid it in the first place. Here are some techniques that can be helpful.

Pay Attention to Your Environment

You must manage your environment to prevent or minimize the symptoms of depression. Play upbeat music, open the curtains and have plenty of lights on, watch comedies, and keep yourself looking good by dressing well and maintaining your hygiene. When you look better, you often feel better. Pretend you have a guest coming over and you want to make things special for him or her. It will help motivate you to straighten up and make sure you have things with which to entertain your guest and make him or her comfortable.

Plants in your home and office are a great idea. Buy or pick flowers and keep them nearby; the good smell and natural beauty will brighten your days.

Get Moving!

The more you do, the more you will want to do. Get out of that bed in the morning. It may be the roughest time of day for you, but force yourself to get going and you may find that you are rolling along after a while. Force yourself every day if you have to. Get mad at the bipolar monster if you have to. Defy the monster.

Exercise boosts endorphins, which elevate mood. The expression "runner's high" refers to the positive feelings runners experience after very fast or very long runs. If you hate to run, join a gym—and make yourself go. If you can't afford to belong to a gym, find exercise television programs and do aerobics along with the instructor.

We recommend outdoor activities like walking, hiking, biking, and fishing. Going to museums and other public places can help get you out of your funk. Happiness is contagious. Hanging around in places where people are laughing and playing are great funk fighters. Even if it is the last thing you feel like doing, get moving and go outside so you can see that there is a great big world out there that you deserve to be a part of.

Red Flag

We should warn you that shopping can be dangerous. Studies show that people who are depressed spend three times more than they spend when they are happy. Sometimes a little "retail therapy" is in order, but be careful that you don't ruin your financial stability in the process.

If hanging out with a bunch of happy people makes you even more depressed, then you are not ready for that. Try hanging out with angry people (who will not be angry at you). It may not be happiness, but anger at least feels alive. Find a cause you can use anger with. Yeah! Kick some butt (metaphorically)! Champion a cause! Advocate for someone who needs it!

Believe it or not, having a pet helps depression. If you don't have the kind of lifestyle that can include a pet, borrow one for the weekend from a friend.

De-Stress

Alternatively, it's okay to chill out, take it slow, and check out for a while. Stress can cause depression or worsen its symptoms. It is very important to learn what causes your stress. Avoid stressors and find ways to minimize any unavoidable stress in your life. Repetitive or constant stress can lead to tension, chronic pain, anxiety, and depression. Complete jerks, money matters, noise, lack of time—it can all get anyone into a funk. Keep a log of your depressed episodes and then try to figure out what triggered each one. Keeping track of them can help you discover patterns in your symptoms and stress levels you were unaware of.

Mental Note

Don't be afraid to cancel or postpone a stressful event if you are not feeling well. Avoidance of triggers is a legitimate way of taking care of your mental health.

When you have to face unavoidable stressors, try choosing times when you are as relaxed and rested as possible. Talking with a trusted friend before dealing with a stressful situation helps some people. Others set aside time to be alone after stressful incidents for rest or meditation.

Write

Put pen to paper and spew out all your fears, troubles, and grievances. Writing makes you articulate your feelings, which in turn tends to objectify your emotions. Documenting what is wrong descriptively often puts your problems into better perspective. Reading your journal entries over a period of time can give you and your therapist insight into your thoughts, feelings, and behavior patterns.

Try to also express yourself through music, art, cooking, crafts, or any other activity that you enjoy so long as it is healthy. Creating things is a therapeutic outlet for most anyone—and sometimes a tasty one at that.

 Red Flag

The absolute worst thing you can do is use alcohol or illicit drugs to cope with stressors. You must process your stress and be kind to yourself to prevent stress from becoming pain or depression. Escaping your stress with substances only allows it to pile up inside you, until its weight is too great to carry—and you experience an episode.

You Are What You Eat

Avoid stimulants like caffeine. Chocolate contains caffeine but is also known to boost serotonin, so if you love it like we do, you might want to just cut back, or get the semi-sweet, and make sure you do not consume it at night when it may keep you awake. Bronchial dilators like psuedoephedrine, found in cold and allergy medications, are stimulants as well. Recent research draws a connection between nicotine addiction and depression. Nicotine is a stimulant and you should avoid it, but if you're a smoker you will probably need help to quit because of the positive feeling smoking provides.

Eat a variety of foods every day, and eat every few hours. This will keep your metabolism high and give you the energy, protein, vitamins, minerals, and fiber you need. Some medications used to treat depression rob you of essential vitamins and minerals, so it is a good idea to take a daily multivitamin along with your meals. Remember, vitamins are dietary *supplements*, not replacements, so you still must eat plenty of vegetables and fruits (preferably raw) and whole grains.

Moderate your intake of fats, especially trans fats (okay to take omega-3 fatty acids), cholesterol, sugars, and salt. Drink lots of water. Don't skip meals, as it will worsen your mood.

Red Flag _____

Look for triggers that may cause overeating. Avoid these triggers and keep plenty of healthy snacks on hand. If you don't keep junk food in your house, you are far less likely to eat it. Always have fresh fruit, yogurt, whole-grain bread, and crackers on hand.

Sleep

Get plenty of sleep. During sleep your brain produces little chemical packages of consciousness for you to use the next day. Sleep is also when most repairs are done throughout your entire body.

Get comfortable pillows and sheets. Keep the bedroom cool, even in the winter. It should be cold enough that you have to get under the covers. Research shows people fall asleep faster when the room is cool and dark. Remove the television from the bedroom so your brain can stop being stimulated and relax.

Mental Note _____

Buy a sound machine. Many manufacturers sell alarm clocks that include different soothing tracks. Ocean waves crashing onto the beach, forest sounds with birds chirping, and rain are commonly offered soothing sounds. They may lull you to sleep, with the added benefit of masking street noise and other potential distractions to your slumber.

By the same token, wake up at a decent hour and start your day. It has been theorized that people with BP have a 25-hour biological clock. They always want to stay up that extra hour. Force yourself to align with the third planet from the sun. Set your biological clock to Earth time and adjust it when it tries to get that extra hour in.

Develop a Sense of Humor

Okay, so last Friday, you made a crack about your boss's bald spot in front of the secretaries in the cafeteria. Now you are depressed and worried about it. If you hadn't been manic, you would have remembered how sensitive he is about that. And now it's time for your annual review and you need this year's bonus to pay off the credit cards you ran up buying rounds for everyone at the bar. What do you say to the boss?

"I'm sorry I cracked a joke about your bald spot the other day"? Nah. I wouldn't say that.

"Are you going to protest my unemployment compensation?" No.

"I'm wondering if you, in your baldness, can be objective about my performance appraisal?" Don't do that.

Maybe this. Before you go in for your performance appraisal, simply acknowledge everything and take responsibility for it. "I guess I was a real ass last Friday. I have to apologize for that."

Humbleness is always a good counter after displaying ego, arrogance, and entitlement. Groveling can sometimes get you points back. Asking how you can make it up might even out the wrinkle. Humorous self-chastisement might assist. Offering a token of peace may help (flowers, for example).

Looking at things with a sense of humor gets you out of yourself. It enables you to see yourself. You have a choice in the way you take life. You can take it seriously or you can take it with a sense of humor, for example. A sense of humor forces you to use that lobe. It forces you to take the lobe out for a spin. Being serious only needs the cognitive thinker, and we all know how serious thoughts can build to catastrophic proportion, worry, and a sense of doom.

Do Something for Other People (or Animals)

Doing something kind for others can really help you feel better. Many people find it emotionally rewarding to help other people, especially children, the elderly, or handicapped individuals. And don't forget our furry (or feathered) friends. Volunteer at your local animal shelter, perhaps to walk the dogs. Additional benefits to dog walking are fresh air and exercise. The enthusiasm, appreciation, and affection from a dog rubs off.

Helping people who are worse off than you puts things into perspective sometimes. You may realize that you don't have it so bad.

The Least You Need to Know

 ◆ Depression can show itself via a variety of symptoms, ranging from anger and anxiety to social withdrawal and lack of personal hygiene.

- Certain factors can cause your bipolar disorder to escalate to the point of suicide; knowing the causes can save your life.

- There are many things you can do to avoid (or lessen) a depressive phase, such as adjusting your sleep cycle and watching your diet.

- Treating bipolar depression may be difficult—there is no magic wand.

Chapter **7**

Other Related Problems

In This Chapter

- ◆ Besides bipolar, what else?
- ◆ Bipolar often looks and acts like obsessive compulsive disorder
- ◆ The connection between BP and weight gain
- ◆ Why can't I sleep?

Bipolar disorder, as we have said, can be exacerbated by other things. It can be provoked by trauma, hormones, street drugs, some prescription medications, and it can also be provoked by other problems such as stress, other mental health problems, and deprivation of sleep. In this chapter, we will look at how bipolar disorder affects other medical conditions and vice versa.

People with BP are almost forced to take good care of themselves because when they fall, they fall big. Take your vitamins, omega-3, get exercise, keep your life as stress-free as possible, have a routine, get enough sleep, and listen to people you trust. Stay out of stressful situations. Select good friends and a good mate. Ah! If we could all just do those things that were good for us!

BP's Effect on Other Medical Conditions

BP's effect on other medical conditions can vary widely depending upon the specific condition involved. Is it diabetes, seasonal-affective disorder, heart problems, attention deficit, arthritis, generalized anxiety disorder, chronic fatigue, hepatitis, gastritis, irritable bowel syndrome, high blood pressure, HIV, cancer, or something else not mentioned yet?

In any of the preceding cases, the medications have to be compatible. They can't be contraindicated (incompatible). Make sure the doctors know all of the medications you are on.

Mental Note _____

In this great age of technology, some drug store computers will spit out a warning if any of the drugs you are taking have an interaction. There are also websites that allow you to enter the drugs you are on and find out if there are any adverse interactions.

You need to be an advocate for yourself. Don't worry—you are bright enough to do it. Yes, some of these medications have side effects. So you might have to ask yourself questions like, "Okay, do I want to feel a little nauseous right after I take my medication, or do I want to have a manic episode and completely destroy my life—drinking, gambling, shopping, and ruining my relationships?" And you may have to choose this every day of your life. You can probably address the nausea, but the police won't forgive that DWI, and the gambling casino is not going to give your money back. They will just give you a number for Gamblers Anonymous.

Let's take a couple of examples to illustrate the types of things that could happen with other medical problems and BP.

Generalized Anxiety Disorder

Let's say the doctor is treating you for generalized anxiety disorder (GAD) with an SSRI medication. In the process of treatment, you have a manic episode and jump out of your second-story window holding an open umbrella to break your fall. Now you are in the hospital with two broken ankles, you can't sleep, and you are worried about losing your job. You are having racing thoughts, and you can't seem to focus. You are worried what the neighbors think about you, and you feel stupid. You think the doctor wants to give you an antipsychotic drug to make you feel "stupider." You might actually welcome that if it stops your mind from racing and the worries from being so intense.

The doctor may give you a mood stabilizer to prevent the SSRI from triggering a manic episode. She may give you olanzapine, which will likely take care of the GAD and the BP. If you have both medical problems, you probably haven't felt or been well since adolescence. These two may be difficult to detect together. If you go to the doctor and say you feel anxiety, she may give you a benzodiazepine (ativan, xanax, klonopin, valium). The benzos can mask your bipolar agitation as well as block the anxiety. It appears to work, but it is only masking the symptoms. If you happen to be a recovering alcoholic or former addict, the benzos may stimulate the addiction center in your brain and you may start using again. Most doctors are not trained in addictions, so he may not realize this could happen. You might frustrate him by telling him you can't take addictive medications, but you need to.

If you have an astute doctor, she may pick up that you have both disorders. Medication is difficult because there are limited choices for treating both conditions. You may end up with olanzapine along with an SSRI, which may treat it very well. Then you may have to deal with a weight gain.

You may want to make sure you have both conditions. GAD almost always has a digestive-system problem like acid reflux, gastritis, colitis, or irritable bowel syndrome associated with it. In the family history, you can usually find a worrywart somewhere (maybe Grandma, who used to have a little drink once in a while for medicinal purposes only). Some of the symptoms of BP and GAD are similar, like the difficulty sleeping and irritability. With GAD, a person can have catastrophic thinking, which could be misinterpreted as the grandiose thinking that would come with mania. The consensus among therapists is that people with GAD are usually artistically creative while people with BP tend to think out of the box.

High Blood Pressure

Let's say you have high blood pressure and you are diagnosed with bipolar disorder. Here's one problem: most of the medications for bipolar disorder tend to have weight gain associated with them, which is likely to make your blood pressure go even higher. The doctor may then add topamax or a glucophage (like metformin) to your medication regimen so that you can contain or even lose weight.

Liver and Kidney Problems

If you have hepatitis C and have been diagnosed with bipolar disorder, make sure the doctor knows this. He won't be able to use medications that flow through the liver.

If you have had kidney problems and the doctor wants to put you on lithium, make sure your doctor knows all about your medical history. Lithium flows through the kidneys. Again, this would be a concern, so you and your doctor should consider alternative medications.

We could show countless examples. This is where a membership in the DBSA (Depression and Bipolar Support Alliance) and NAMI (National Alliance on Mental Illness) would be important because you are likely to find someone with the same set of problems who can tell you what has worked for them. Both DBSA and NAMI have online chats. Ah, technology!

Obsessive Compulsive Disorder

In one study, 20 percent of people with bipolar disorder had OCD. This author has trouble believing that statistic because there is sometimes an obsessiveness that appears with mania that is *not* OCD. OCD can actually be a "manic side-symptom," so a mood stabilizer may address it. If that doesn't work, you can augment with ERP (exposure and response prevention), a non-medication therapy that seems to help in many cases and is not known to make bipolar disorder worse.

To recap: OCD is fear-driven. The typical OCD obsessions are hand washing, checking the stove multiple times, locking the door multiple times, making up rituals to prevent catastrophes, counting certain objects, or counting to certain numbers. If you ask the person with the obsession what would happen if they didn't do what they were doing and they said, "I wouldn't like it," then that is probably not OCD. It is probably an obsession driven by mania (anxiety mania) that will diminish with a mood stabilizer or other bipolar medication.

Since most OCD medication (usually SSRIs) can make BP worse, it is advisable to check and make sure it is a true case of OCD. The right medication, however, can lower your bipolar-caused symptoms of OCD. For example, one young woman had an obsession with a rock star. It wasn't a normal obsession. Her family did not enjoy her company at dinner and her girlfriends didn't want to be around her because all she did was talk about this rock star incessantly. The family was a moral family, but this girl told her father, "Dad, if he ever wanted me, you know, I'd have to let him have me." Whoa! Not a good thing to say to your Dad. It showed lack of insight.

Eventually Dad took her to a psychiatrist and the doctor put her on OCD medication. It didn't put a dent in the OCD and actually made the obsessive thinking worse, so the doctor raised the dosage. That actually made it worse, again. Her Dad took her for a second opinion and the other psychiatrist put her on divalproex sodium (bipolar medication). The obsession about the rock star diminished slowly. After a week, her friends were back and she could keep quiet about the rock star. The next week her company was actually enjoyed by her family. The week after that, she said she still thought about the rock star, but it was just fleeting thoughts. A few weeks into the medication and she said, "I don't know what I ever saw in him."

What was that? The second psychiatrist had a theory that it was a form of mania. The hypersexuality was directed at a safe source (it was unlikely she was ever going to be with the rock star). The racing thoughts were directed at one thing (better than being dispersed with all kinds of thoughts all over the place). She had the talkativeness with a pressure to keep talking.

Was it bipolar? Who cares? The divalproex sodium fixed it. There are some things that are not in the DSM-IV yet. The description of a bipolar child is not in there and neither is the description of a bipolar adolescent. If you thought the DSM-IV was a bible, you are mistaken. Why do you think they call it the DSM-IV? The DSM-V is scheduled to be out in 2012. I am not criticizing the DSM; it's a valuable tool, used in many other countries. But it has always been a work in progress. The moment it becomes a bible is when we stop learning about mental illness. There should always be room for more discoveries in the DSM.

Sleep Deprivation

One of the main problems with bipolar disorder is that it affects sleep. The major symptoms you see with delusions and psychosis are due in large part to a lack of sleep. Mania cuts off the communication between the mind and body (just like taking amphetamines) so the person is full of "energy." Another form of mania feels like anxiety (which is probably physical agitation) and stimulates the worry, the magnification of feelings, and the feeling of not wanting to be in your own skin. The lack of sleep compounds things to an exponential degree. The other mania is the angry mania (it's actually rage) or "irritability" (a little suppressed rage).

You can demonstrate mania by giving people amphetamines over a few weeks, which is thought to duplicate the chemical imbalance of mania. Initially most people will get high (euphoric mania), but some won't. Some people will say they feel "anxiety," but that is not possible. They are just having a physiological reaction to the pill.

I might go to a therapist if I had anxiety. Maybe it would come out that I felt anxiety around my father. There is no such psychological feeling as anxiety. Anxiety is usually the result of a combination of unsorted and unresolved feelings. I might realize through talk-therapy that I was afraid of my father and angry with my father. It would be like two hoses pointed at each other and you would have that watery mess in the middle that we call anxiety. So the next time I was with my father, I might feel the anger and feel the fear, but I wouldn't feel the anxiety.

When you give someone amphetamines and they feel "anxiety," it's probably not anxiety even though it feels exactly like anxiety. It has to be agitation. A lot of people with bipolar disorder are used to agitation. You may see them shaking their foot or tapping. We call it *hypervigilance*. I realize that I have mentioned this before, but it is extremely important information and could save someone's life.

Any human being would be very debilitated with lack of sleep. Any of us could become psychotic from no sleep, and see things that weren't there, and hear voices that seemed exterior to ourselves. This is usually the case with a chronic bipolar disorder where sleep was lacking. So the bipolar disorder causes a lack of sleep—and then the sleep deprivation causes those major symptoms. Do you see why sleep is extremely important?

It's true that one could have such a chemical imbalance that they could become psychotic. That would be like someone taking way too many amphetamines at once. However, the delusions and psychosis usually come from the sleep deprivation. And, of course, there *is* a chemical imbalance.

When a person with BP is put on medication during their "no-sleep" cycle, they will most likely become tired and lethargic. It's not the medication's fault! Most of these medications work much better after the person has had enough rest. You can't expect to lose sleep for days or weeks at a time and not have some aftermath. The body is wiped out. The brain probably lacks serotonin, which means that melatonin is the rule of the brain roost. You can expect to hibernate for a while after a manic episode. Your brain chemicals have to rebalance and your body has to rest. It would only be natural. There is no such thing as having a full-blown manic episode over the weekend, getting treated, and then showing up for work on Monday all chipper.

What should you do about this? Sleep.

Weight Issues

Here we go. This is a tough subject. Most bipolar medications cause a person to gain weight. We have to inundate the body with so much medication to break the blood-brain barrier that it causes metabolism problems (meaning weight gain).

So here we have Ms. BP Extraordinaire, who is coming down from a manic high. She hasn't eaten in a week because mania can suppress appetite. Her lobe isn't functioning because of the mania and she has no insight, foresight, or hindsight. She still has the ego, arrogance, and entitlement that the mania gave her and it hasn't subsided yet. She stands there in her yellow spiked hair and her colorful "threads," beginning to realize that she needs treatment because she lost her beloved boyfriend after he found out she was cheating on him with two other guys. Her bipolar disorder is confirmed when she goes in to see the psychiatrist and he wants to put her on medication. Her first question is, "Is this going to make me gain weight?" He says it is likely that it will. She refuses treatment and out the door she goes to ruin the rest of her life.

This story is not to make fun of her or to blame her. This is a scenario that happens all the time. First of all, she has no insight. BP took her lobe off-line. She has ego, arrogance, and entitlement. This is *not* any indication of a personality problem. One of the prejudices that people with BP encounter is that they may be viewed as someone who is willingly egotistical, arrogant, and has a sense of entitlement. She may be the most considerate person you would ever meet when she is not manic. The real problem is: how do we get this good hearted, wonderful person to take her meds, so that she can manifest the person she really is?

Most likely, we will have to wait until she crashes into a depression and then doesn't care about the weight. Some people will go on the meds but "play" with them because of the weight gain. She will take less than she is supposed to. She may go too far (with no insight) and bang! Here come ego, arrogance, and entitlement again. If she is not so outgoing, she may become passive aggressive, stubborn, and say yes to everyone and then do what she wants (with no insight).

On the other hand, you might have a person who has hit bottom and has every intention of taking the medication. This person gains weight. Some people gain a lot of weight. If we could break the blood-brain barrier with a little bit of lithium or a little bit of any bipolar medication, there wouldn't be the weight gain, the overworked kidneys, and the overworked livers. If we could find a way to automatically shoot a little bit of medication in the brain to keep the chemical balance, the person wouldn't have to remember to take their meds.

In the meantime, we have to try to solve the weight problems with other medications like topiramate or metformin. Topiramate is used for bipolar disorder, but the consensus is that it doesn't totally do the job. A person may have ups and downs on topiramate, but it is used with other medications to keep the weight gain down. Another emerging medication is Glucophage. This is used with diabetics, but can be used along with bipolar medication to prevent diabetes and lessen the weight gain. It has not yet been formally presented to the FDA in a double-blind study to be used with bipolar medications, but you will find small studies on the Internet that say it helps and others that say it has some effect on some people.

There are some medications with minimal weight gain and there are scales that indicate the amount of weight gain for each medication. For example, you will gain the least amount of weight of any of the antipsychotics on aripiprazole. Some of the medications may require you to make an extra trip to the gym every week or run an extra mile. With bipolar disorder your choices are all a shade of gray. There is hardly any perfect solution yet. Pick the lightest shade of gray.

The Least You Need to Know

- ◆ If you are taking medications for another condition, you need to choose your BP meds carefully.

- ◆ It's very important to make sure your doctor is aware of your medical history and any current health problems you have, so he or she can chart the best course of treatment for your bipolar disorder.

- ◆ Bipolar both causes and is exacerbated by sleeplessness. Try to get your rest no matter what.

- ◆ Many bipolar medications will cause weight gain. There are no perfect solutions, but the side effects are still better than the disease.

Chapter 8

When Symptoms Get Serious

In This Chapter

- ◆ Common early warning signs
- ◆ Suicide red flags
- ◆ Deciding whether to seek help—and when

Living with the routine day-to-day symptoms of BP can be difficult enough. More intense symptoms are not to be taken lightly. Sometimes BP can cause new, scary symptoms; sometimes something in your system goes awry and your usual symptoms suddenly escalate to dangerous levels.

One of the biggest problems is that you may be unaware that these symptoms are coming from an imbalance of dopamine. You may experience these symptoms without the benefit of "seeing" what is happening. That is when the people who know you can come in handy. They may be able to "see" if there is anything different about the way you are thinking.

Major Red Flags

Everyone's BP symptoms are different, so you (or those closest to you) are probably the best judge of the early warning signs that something is off. You should closely monitor any noticeable change from your normal condition or behavior, but there are some clear-cut signals of a major problem (or one that might be brewing under the surface).

Severe Mood Swings or Rapid Cycling

One of the most common early red flags is a period of drastic mood swings or rapid cycling. (See Chapter 3 for an explanation of rapid cycling.) This can be tricky to identify, because you may attribute your mood swings to things in your environment and your explanation may be good enough to sound convincing to others (and even yourself).

In fact, something may have happened to trigger your symptoms. You may be magnifying things in your environment. The mood swings may even be a part of your normal pattern, especially if your moods have not been well-controlled lately. If you have hurt the feelings of someone who is not particularly oversensitive, that might be a sign that you are having mood swings. If you find yourself abusing substances or "adjusting" your medication because you think you know better than your doctor, that could be a sign something is wrong. If you end up with extra medication, it is a clear sign you have not taken it when you are supposed to. Inability to stop yourself from talking can be a sign.

Major Changes in Sleep Habits

When things are not as they should be, one of the first signs is often sleeping too much (depression) or sleeping very little (mania). Mania, in its various forms, is like taking amphetamines. If you are clearly manic, you may not feel that you need sleep and feel fine with a small amount. If you are anxious and having racing thoughts, a few different things could be happening:

- ◆ You feel exhausted yet energized, and you can't seem to turn it off.

- ◆ You are irritable or angry and can't stop thinking about things that make you angry.

- ◆ An environmental difficulty has you truly concerned and is triggering your BP.

Change in Eating Habits

Be on the lookout for any noticeable change in your appetite or eating patterns. Usually, this involves loss of appetite or lack of interest in food, although some people gorge on food, especially if they tend to be emotional eaters. Overeating often occurs during the depressive phase.

Sometimes a person with BP is misdiagnosed with anorexia. Mania can suppress appetite. Along with that, mania is almost always accompanied by a lack of sleep, which may not be present in anorexia. In other types of mania, eating is compulsive and the experience of the taste of food is the goal. You may crave certain tastes or crave crunchy things if angry-manic. But most people who are manic eat less than normal.

Use of Alcohol or Drugs

People with bipolar disorder are much more likely to use drugs or alcohol, especially if they aren't following a good routine of medication and/or therapy. The drug of choice can be …

- An upper (if depression is present) like cocaine, meth, amphetamines, caffeine, Ritalin, or Adderall.

- A downer (if one's thoughts are racing and there is a feeling of being all over the place) like alcohol, Xanax, heroin, or any of the benzodiazepines.

- Marijuana (for mood swings). Ecstasy or LSD may also be used to switch moods.

The reason for the substance abuse is usually in part to feel better. One of the questions to ask yourself is, "Am I doing this to feel better or to get high?"

If you are doing it to feel better, it is more likely to be your BP driving you to abuse the substance. If you are doing it to get high, it is more likely your addictive behavior. Either way, your BP stability is at stake. And yes, you could be doing it to get high *and* to feel better, in which case it is partially BP and partially addictive behavior.

 Red Flag

Substance abuse can be especially dangerous for bipolar patients who are taking medication. Medications can have a serious negative interaction when combined with alcohol and/or other drugs. For example, if you are on lithium and drink lots of beer, it could seriously affect your kidneys and metabolic system.

Disinterest in Things That Are Important to You

If you suddenly become apathetic about things that you normally care a lot about, this should make you take notice. If others start asking you why you are no longer interested in certain things, it's time to ask yourself why. Did you switch your interest to something else, or have you just stopped being interested in things in general? Have you become a couch potato? Has your sex drive dropped? A disinterest in activities that were once pleasurable is a distinct sign of depression.

Withdrawal or Isolation

This can go hand-in-hand with the sudden disinterest in things (or people) you normally care about. If you find yourself wanting to withdraw or hide from the world, alert your doctor and take action to nip this in the bud. It can be very tempting to retreat to bed and hide under the covers, but that is actually the worst thing you can do. You will only get increasingly depressed and likely end up trapped in a downward spiral. Call a trusted friend, make plans, and force yourself to keep the commitment.

Relationship Troubles

This is one of those chicken-and-egg things. Any unusual stress (such as the kind that accompanies relationship troubles) can trigger a downward spiral. Conversely, if you are already headed for trouble, you will often act out against the people closest to you, resulting in strained—or broken—relationships.

No matter in which order it happens, you need to be aware that relationship drama can trigger and/or signal problems with your psychological state. It's time to go to a trusted friend, therapist, or close relative and check your perceptions on a troubled relationship.

Delusions, Hallucinations, and Hearing Things

If you start having any kind of *hallucinations* or begin to hear sounds or voices that aren't really there, this is a serious red flag. *Delusions*—including delusions of grandeur (where you think you're rich, famous, really powerful, or important)—have occurred with bipolar disorder, especially during manic phases. If you are losing sleep and start hearing voices or having peripheral hallucinations, it is time to get help before you totally lose it. Chances are that your sleep pattern has not been good and you are experiencing severe sleep deprivation.

Your brain chemicals could be so unbalanced that you are on your way to becoming psychotic. If you have any sense of yourself left, it is time to ask (beg, scream, yell) for help. The challenge, of course, is that when you are experiencing these episodes, it can be tough for you to determine what's real and what isn't. You might need to rely on your loved ones to alert you when things don't appear normal.

def•i•ni•tion

Hallucinations are a perception in the absence of a stimulus. In a visual hallucination, you might see an angel rise up from the floor and float near the ceiling. In an auditory hallucination, you might hear, for example, a voice telling you to hurt yourself. There can also be tactile or olfactory hallucinations, where you feel or smell something that isn't really there.

Delusions are incorrect beliefs that occur in the context of many pathological states (both physical and mental). However, they are particularly diagnostic of severe bipolar mania and chronic or acute lack of sleep. A mild delusion is thinking that people are talking about you when they are not. A major delusion is thinking you are appointed by God to sweep the sidewalks on your street.

Social Anxiety or Extreme Nervousness

As someone with BP, you should be concerned if you are suddenly struck with social anxiety or constant worry and nervousness. If you find yourself becoming tense just thinking about interacting with other people, or if you experience any type of panic attack, you should consult your doctor right away. If you have bipolar disorder, it could be that you missed your medication or took it twice. If you are on an antipsychotic, it could be that you are experiencing restlessness related to the medication. The keywords here are "suddenly struck" rather than a low-level anxiety. Either way, you need to inform your doctor, but a major bout of anxiety suggests that you should call the doctor sooner rather than later.

Taking Extreme Risks

People who are in a manic phase often feel invincible or fail to consider the consequences of their actions. As a result, they may take extreme risks or engage in dangerous behavior. If you notice that people are trying to warn you about this, you need to stop and think about what you are doing and why. Ask your loved ones to keep a lookout for this type of behavior.

Some people with BP have gambled away their life savings, contracted sexually transmitted diseases, been arrested for illegal drugs, and suffered other negative consequences of their risky behaviors. If you find yourself leaning toward doing things like this, get help right away. By the time you actually do these things, you may feel manic invincibility and ego. By then, it may be too late.

Suicidal Signs

Any intentions of suicide or violence toward others warrant immediate attention and concern. A thought is one thing, but an intention contains the readiness to go through with the violent act. If you have a plan to commit suicide or harm another person, it is time to get help.

> **Research Says**
>
> The suicide rate for people with bipolar disorder is almost 20 percent. When you take into account people with undiagnosed BP, it is believed that the rate is closer to 25 percent. People with BP who commit suicide usually do it in the first two years after onset. Women with BP are at a greater risk of committing suicide than men.

One of the biggest concerns for anyone with bipolar disorder is the risk of suicide or attempted suicide. You need to be very conscientious of even the tiniest little sign that you're starting to feel suicidal. The people around you (friends and family and your treatment professionals) should stay alert for any sign that you may be feeling suicidal. Suicide is a permanent solution to a temporary problem—a temporary problem that may seem inescapable and permanent because your mind is stuck.

Talking or Thinking About Suicide

This is an obvious one. If you are thinking about hurting yourself or talking about suicide, that's a clear signal that you need immediate help. You (or your doctor) should talk with your loved ones to stress the importance of taking any suicidal actions, threats, or even casual jokes seriously. Many grief-stricken survivors regret that they didn't recognize or act upon signs of distress in a suicidal person.

It's possible your loved ones may not take your threats seriously, especially if you couch them in a joking manner. Or they may think you are just trying to get attention (especially if you've done drastic things to seek attention in the past). And perhaps you don't seriously intend to take your life, but any mention or thought of suicide is a cry for help, and your loved ones need to be aware of that.

You may want to verbalize this either way. For example, you might say, "I feel like I want to die. I am not going to do anything to cause it. I just want you to know how bad I feel."

If you have thought of a plan, you may want to say that: "I feel like getting Dad's gun and shooting myself." Then steps can be taken to help you. Chances are that you just want to stop the pain, that you don't know how, and that it seems to go on forever. You have nothing to lose by asking for help. If you don't get help the first time you ask, ask someone else or call your doctor. Your doctor will respond. If you don't have a doctor, call the emergency room or the police. They are trained to respond.

Severe Isolation, Withdrawal, or Avoidance

As we mentioned earlier in this chapter, people in a depressed state often try to hide from the world and avoid other people. If you have isolated yourself from those around you—or have a strong urge to do so—that is cause for concern. Likewise, any type of withdrawal or avoidance that disrupts your daily routine (say, you don't even want to get out of bed, or you miss work or other obligations) is a serious red flag.

This is not uncommon for people with BP. It could be a sign that your medication needs adjusting or that you just need to get out and get moving even if you don't want to. Chances are that once you get going, you will be okay. Mornings are not the best time of the day for many people with BP. Oh sure, you will get some morning people, but many are not.

People with BP have a tendency to think that *they* are the reason they feel the way they do and that they are messing up their lives. They feel they can't change. If you are doing this, step back from that and look at yourself! It's the physiological imbalance causing (triggering) negative thoughts, negative feelings, and negative "tudes" (attitudes). It's just a tude. You have had other tudes.

Self-Injury

People who are contemplating suicide may do a trial run or start out with nonfatal types of self-injury, in order to "work their way up" to taking that permanent step. If you find yourself causing any type of self-injury, such as cutting or burning yourself— or even if you just get the urge to do this—immediate action is warranted.

Some people just want to feel better and do drastic things to achieve that. Some people have no intention of committing suicide, but cutting or burning themselves

Red Flag _____

Even if it's not a precursor to a suicide attempt, any type of self-injury or physically dangerous behavior is a sign that you need immediate help.

releases endorphins and helps relieve them from their mental anguish. These actions are an indication of the need to see a therapist who is experienced in this sort of situation.

Feelings of desperation can come from the bipolar disorder itself, a psychological problem, or both. The best bet is to see a doctor and a therapist or psychologist.

Risk-Taking and Destructive Actions

Sometimes, people who are suicidal prefer to take a passive approach—they want to stop living, but they can't or won't hurt themselves. So, they try to make it likely that someone—or something—else will do it for them. This means they take extraordinary risks or engage in destructive behavior (say, walking on the edge of a steep cliff, or maybe just provoking a fight with a much bigger person) and hope they get the desired result.

If you find yourself doing this, you need to realize that it is just as serious a suicide attempt as a more deliberate approach.

When to Call for Help

If you or your loved ones notice any of the red flags mentioned in this chapter, you should call your doctor right away. However, there are times when you need immediate help—a call to 911 or a trip to the ER or another treatment facility. Here are a few signs that you need help right now:

- You have become physically violent toward someone else (or attempted to do so).

- You are about to hurt yourself or have already done so.

- You experience any type of psychotic episodes: hallucinations, hearing things, blackouts, or other occurrences where you don't seem to be in touch with reality.

- You have suffered physical harm as a result of your manic or depressive phases (for example, you're feeling faint because you have gone too long without eating).

A Final Important Note

You (or your loved ones) may be hesitant to seek emergency treatment for fear of seeming overdramatic. Or perhaps you are unsure if your symptoms are really as serious as they seem, or you think you can hold out until your regularly scheduled appointment.

Our advice—and we can't stress this enough—is to seek help right away whenever you have the slightest inclination that things might be serious or heading that way. If you have BP, your doctors would much rather that you err on the side of caution. Things can go downhill quickly, so the sooner you act on the first sign of trouble, the better. Ideally, you will catch an impending problem while it's still in the early stages, when it can be treated much more easily.

Bottom line: it's better to be safe than sorry. We're not trying to be overdramatic or frighten you, but in the case of a bipolar person who might be taking a wrong turn, seeking immediate help can often be the difference between life and death. It can be the difference between taking preventative measures or finding yourself in a bipolar typhoon.

The Least You Need to Know

◆ Changes in appetite, sleep patterns, socialization, and daily routines can be early warning signs of a bigger problem down the line.

◆ If you suffer hallucinations, hear voices or other nonexistent sounds, or have the urge to hurt yourself or someone else, you need to get immediate help.

◆ If you're concerned about troubling signs you see in yourself or a loved one—even if you're not sure the sign is something serious—consult a professional or seek treatment right away, just to be on the safe side.

9

Bipolar Disorder in Young People

In This Chapter

- ◆ How BP affects kids differently than it does adults
- ◆ The difficulty of diagnosis in young people
- ◆ Specific challenges of using BP meds for kids

An increasing number of children and teenagers are being diagnosed with bipolar disorder. This condition can take its toll on the young person, who is already dealing with myriad challenges of growing up, but it can also be draining for the entire family.

The Basics of Bipolar Disorder in Kids and Teens

While some concerns and symptoms of BP are universal (regardless of age), some aspects of the disorder are different in young people. Before we get into that, though, let's look at how common BP is in young people—and how challenging it can be to diagnose these younger patients.

Statistics

It's tough to pinpoint the exact number of young people who have bipolar disorder, as they are often undiagnosed or misdiagnosed. There are also trends that contribute to the number of diagnoses, as shown by Dr. Gransee in Chapter 22. Many kids who have been diagnosed with ADD, ADHD, conduct disorder, or oppositional defiant disorder may actually suffer from BP. And the more different diagnoses a child has, the more likely it is that he actually suffers from BP. One of the most consistent things about bipolar disorder is that it is inconsistent in children.

Most statistics involving bipolar children are only rough estimates, given the widespread belief that the disorder is much more common among young people than official figures indicate. The American Academy of Child and Adolescent Psychiatry has estimated that up to one third of the 3.4 million children and adolescents who have been diagnosed with depression in the United States may actually be suffering from bipolar disorder.

One author evaluated 150 children in a high-risk group in Pennsylvania in 1993 and diagnosed 6 percent with bipolar disorder who had been previously diagnosed with ADHD. These children came from biological parents who were incarcerated, had mental health problems, who had abandoned them, or were destitute. Ninety-three percent of bipolar kids meet the criteria for a diagnosis of ADHD. However, psychostimulants, which are commonly prescribed to treat ADHD, can make these children psychotic, suicidal, or homicidal. The author feels that ADHD and bipolar disorder are currently overdiagnosed.

On one hand there are probably still children who are bipolar and missed. On the other hand, the disorder has become so popular that kids are being diagnosed who do not actually meet the full criteria. Just because a kid is angry and he can't sleep doesn't mean he has bipolar disorder. Just because he is unruly and the medication calms him down doesn't necessarily mean the kid is bipolar. We need to be more certain before we treat a child with psychotropic medication. We also need more expertise when we see a child who's been diagnosed with all sorts of things that come and go (oppositional defiance, conduct disorder, anxiety, Asperger's, learning disabilities, ADHD, and so on). The child may just have bipolar disorder, which pops out every so often with a bipolar symptom or two, trying to "fly under the radar" of fully waking up the bipolar monster.

Bipolar disorder can cause a child to appear as if he has ADHD. A bipolar child's developing executive functions may engage and then go off-line. This may cause the child to appear as if he *temporarily* has ADHD, conduct disorder, oppositional defiant disorder, or even a learning disability. But conduct disorder is consistent. ADHD is consistent. If a child seems to have conduct disorder one day and the next day he shows remorse and empathy, he does not have conduct disorder. If he doesn't see the context of a situation and can't focus one day, but is able to focus the next day, he does not have ADHD. Again, the most consistent thing about BP is that it is inconsistent in children.

Research Says
The Child and Adolescent Bipolar Foundation has estimated that as many as 15 percent of kids diagnosed with ADHD may actually have bipolar disorder.

Diagnosis Difficulties

As we've said, it can be difficult to correctly diagnose a young person who may be suffering from BP. The BP diagnosis guidelines medical professionals traditionally use (as outlined in the DSM-IV) don't differentiate by age. The DSM-IV's one-size-fits-all approach can be a problem, because BP often exhibits itself differently in kids than it does in adults.

Plus, it can be tough to figure out which of a young person's "symptoms" are simply normal childhood or teenage phases, and which are something more serious. For example, one sign of bipolar disorder can be erratic sleep patterns. But many young people—especially babies and toddlers and busy teens—have unusual sleep patterns, and they don't all have bipolar disorder.

The teen years can be especially challenging when it comes to making a conclusive BP diagnosis. As anyone who has ever parented (or simply interacted with) a teenager can attest, they can be moody for no physical reason at all. Then there are the "normal" periods of depression and anxiety that many teens experience. Unlike BP-caused moods, these depressions are often situational—meaning they're triggered by something (say, a breakup with a boyfriend or a disappointing experience).

The adult criteria for BP indicates that certain symptoms must have a duration of one week or more. These include grandiosity, less need for sleep, abnormal talkativeness, racing thoughts, and pursuing high-risk, goal-oriented endeavors. This longer duration makes sense for diagnosing adults, but is less likely to occur in children. Children are rapid cyclers. They don't have a straight week of anything. Adolescents are in between adults and children. They usually don't have five days of anything, either.

Bipolar children, being rapid cyclers, may have their moods go up and down a couple times a day. A child's depression may not look like depression. It may look like irritability or boredom. During a manic moment, you will probably notice some grandiosity. This is different from ADHD kids.

There is another way you can see the difference between an ADHD kid and a bipolar kid. If an ADHD kid has a bad dream in which someone is chasing him with a knife, he will usually wake up before he is stabbed. A bipolar kid is likely to sleep through the stabbing and gore. Bipolar kids can have fairly morbid dreams.

An ADHD kid (and most other kids) can usually sustain a temper tantrum for 12 to 20 minutes, followed by exhaustion. A bipolar kid can have a tantrum lasting well beyond a half hour, and maybe all afternoon. It seems that once a bipolar child's adrenaline is triggered, it keeps looping in what can look like a never-ending episode. It is not a willful tantrum after a while. You can see in the child's eyes that he wants to stop but can't get off it. He may reach out and want comfort, at the same time still tantruming.

Red Flag

Any child or teen who exhibits behavior of serious concern—substance abuse, violence, suicidal threats or actions, or excessively risky behavior—should be evaluated by a mental health professional. If bipolar disorder is a concern (for instance, if it runs in the family), make sure the professional is trained to recognize it.

Mental Note

Many pediatricians lack the training or expertise to diagnose or treat bipolar disorder. If you suspect your child has symptoms, seek a consultation with a mental health professional—preferably one who specializes in treating children and is trained in bipolar disorder.

If an ADHD kid or a child with PTSD doesn't sleep the normal number of hours for his age, he will be tired the next day. A bipolar kid may get very little sleep and not feel tired the next day.

Another sign of BP is risk-taking behavior during manic stages. But how many teens do you know who engage in risky behavior, at least occasionally? Chances are, quite a few.

Teens and preteens also aren't very forthcoming about their feelings and innermost thoughts (at least to adults), which can add to the difficulty of getting a proper diagnosis. It is always a good idea for parents to talk to their child's therapist and give feedback before or after the child sees the therapist.

There is good information on bipolar children on the Child and Adolescent Bipolar Foundation website (www.bpkids.org) and in *The Bipolar Child*, by Demitri Papolos and Janice Papolos. These resources will help you determine the possibility of BP in your child. But keep in mind that no single symptom alone makes a diagnosis.

Specific Age Groups

The symptoms and concerns related to BP vary according to a child's age. In the next few sections, we will look at specific issues connected to particular age groups.

Children

In children (up to age 10 or so), BP can be tricky to spot. This is especially true with kids of preschool age or younger. Many non-BP kids can be clingy, hyper, irritable, and erratic sleepers—all symptoms that can also signify a bipolar condition. Parents need to be alert for things like rapid mood swings, major or ongoing periods of depression, sudden periods of isolation and anxiety, and abnormal risky or manic behavior. Night terrors and talkativeness with grandiosity are two other common traits of bipolar children, although these (especially night terrors) can also occur in kids without BP. Obviously, any mention of suicide or attempts to cause self-injury warrant immediate attention.

> **Mental Note**
>
> Your child's teacher can often provide valuable insight that can help your doctor reach—or rule out—a BP diagnosis. For example, if your child acts a bit withdrawn at home but socializes well with his or her classmates, this may mean he's just acting like a normal teen who needs space from his parents. If, on the other hand, the teacher says your child is moody, or has fits of unstoppable giggling, or is defiant at times, these symptoms together could mean something more. Again, no one or two things mean a child has bipolar disorder. But an accumulation of several factors may indicate a need for further follow-up.

Preteens

Consensus among mental health professionals is that the onset of bipolar disorder happens in adolescence for most people. During the preteen years, many parents first start to notice BP-related symptoms in their children. That's partly because a child of this age is experiencing incredible physical, psychological, and emotional changes and growth—which can often aggravate existing BP symptoms or serve as a catalyst for bipolar behaviors. A case of bipolar disorder that had been dormant will often become more obvious when puberty hits and a whole new batch of hormones and chemicals are added to the mix.

Unlike their younger counterparts, preteens have the verbal skills and maturity to assess and verbalize their moods and feelings. However, that doesn't mean they *want* to. While some kids this age are willing to communicate with parents (and doctors), others can be very tight-lipped. Proceed cautiously, and tailor your approach to your child's personality. The key is to find out how the child is feeling without coming across like an interrogator.

Red Flag

It's important for both parents to be on the same page when it comes to the treatment and parenting of their bipolar child. For one thing, doctors are often reluctant to pursue a specific course of treatment if one parent opposes it. The child may sense the parents' conflicts, which will only add to the child's stressed emotional state.

Teenagers

Teenagers are in between being a child and an adult. Their symptoms are unlikely to last a week or more. They may exhibit more specific symptoms than children, but these may switch easily. One morning a teenager's life is over because the person she loved is going out with someone else. But the afternoon may bring joy and happiness because the person she *really* wanted to go out with called her.

Combined with the typical teenage pressures (school, friends, peer pressure, and so on), bipolar symptoms can often seem overwhelming. That's why it's critical for parents to make sure their bipolar (or potentially bipolar) teen gets proper treatment. Parents need to be alert for the first signs of trouble. Bipolar teens can quickly sink into a deep depression and find themselves unable to cope or handle everyday life. Suicide, substance abuse, and high-risk behavior are common threats to BP teens, and their loved ones need to be diligent about watching for red flags.

Puberty's Effect on Bipolar

Everyone knows that puberty is a time of intense change and growth for young people. Their bodies go through a lot of complex processes—physically, mentally, and emotionally. Not surprisingly, this can be a rough time for a bipolar child. All of the chemical reactions and hormonal changes can wreak havoc on a bipolar child's system. New symptoms may crop up, old ones may seem to disappear, and meds can begin to work totally differently than they did just a short time ago.

A parent has to ask internal questions like, "Is this mania I'm seeing, or is this child showing disrespect?" If it is disrespect, there should be consequences. If it is angry mania, there is no point in punishing a child for something he has no control over. If the brain is connected directly to the tongue in a temporary "Tourette's" moment, let it go.

If there is a sibling that wonders why there is no consequences for his behavior, simply tell the sibling, "He can't help it. You can, so there would be consequences. When he can help it, there will be consequences for him, too." Children usually have more acceptance than adults, so they might be okay with this. If a bipolar child starts using his disorder as an excuse, it may be time to intervene. When you find that your bipolar son puts a frog in his sister's bed and then says, "I couldn't help it. I'm bipolar!" Uh, no. It's time for some consequences!

Sleep

Everyone needs to get proper sleep, but it's especially important for young people with bipolar disorder. Lack of sleep can trigger or worsen bipolar symptoms, and it can also cause medications to work less effectively.

Conversely, an existing or escalating problem often exhibits itself as a change in sleep habits—usually going longer than normal (perhaps even several days) with little or no sleep.

Parents should monitor sleep habits closely. They may be the most significant causal element in triggering an episode. Sleep is also the most significant symptom when an episode has been triggered by something else. Lack of sleep can cause BP symptoms or be the result of BP emerging. Sleep starts it or compounds the problem. As such, it is the one symptom/cause to address first. Rarely, a person can have bipolar disorder without a sleep problem.

Medications

For parents of bipolar children, medication—and all of the issues surrounding it—can be one of the most troubling aspects of their children's treatment plans. Many parents are hesitant to put their kids on medication—and rightly so. Most of the meds used to treat BP are strong, powerful, serious drugs, and parents need to give serious thought to what their children take.

The following stories show a variety of medication decisions that informed parents have made.

Testimonial from an informed mother in Maryland of an adolescent boy:

> *We decided to slowly wean our son from his antipsychotic medication. He was stable. We know that bipolar disorder is episodic, so we decided to watch him closely and try to create an environment where he wouldn't be triggered. The episode that he had was triggered by SSRI antidepressants. We have switched to an antidepressant that is not known to cause mania. We asked the doctor for some BP medication to keep on hand. We can give him this medication if he has another episode and it will keep him somewhat stable until he can see his psychiatrist. He is taking lamotrigine, which we understand is a low-level antidepressant and a preventative for bipolar episodes. He is also getting omega-3 fish oil, which the National Institute of Mental Health (NIMH) says is a preventative. He is seeing a therapist who specializes in social rhythm therapy, which is a hybrid therapy for BP.*

A mother in Berks County, Pennsylvania, of a feisty adolescent girl:

> *We are keeping our daughter on her medication. She has three different medications. She has had three episodes and tried to cut her wrists twice. She almost died in one attempt. She refuses to attend a bipolar group. She would not take her medication every day unless we were here to give it to her and sometimes talk her into it. We have threatened to drive her to a facility in Philadelphia if she doesn't take the medication. We feel she is at risk, and until that changes, this is the regimen we have chosen for her. She likes her psychiatrist but also gives him a hard time.*

A mother from Sonoma County, California:

> *We have taken our son off medication a few times. He ends up acting out at school, and the school will not allow him to attend if he is going to distract other children and defy the teachers. When he is on his medication, he doesn't act up and he is able to make friends. If we take him off his meds, he won't feel good about himself and he will be labeled a behavior problem. We would rather take the risk on the medication and have him grow up in a normal school setting and have friends and self-esteem.*

A mother from Reading, Pennsylvania:

> *We took our daughter to a therapist, whom she loves. We have worked with the psychiatrist to use the minimal amount of medication. Her sleep medication seems the most important. She takes a low dose of risperidone at night; otherwise she is up in the wee hours of the morning and ends up having mood swings and becoming belligerent the next day. She doesn't like herself acting that way (we can tell), but she can't seem to help it.*

We became aware of her problem after school officials told us she was eroticized. The school suspected her father of molesting her. Then a psychiatrist diagnosed her with BP and said she was just hypersexual because of BP and didn't show signs of knowledge with her sexual acting out. Heck of a way to find out your kid has bipolar disorder! She is adopted, and we found out that her biological mother has bipolar disorder and used drugs while pregnant.

All of the preceding treatment plans seem appropriate for the circumstances. When circumstances change, plans should, too. It is very difficult to raise a bipolar child. One has to know the disorder well enough to know when to hold the parent card and when to hold the nursing card.

Medications Affect Kids Differently

Many medications commonly used to treat bipolar adults are generally not used, or used only as a last resort, for bipolar children. Only a handful of bipolar meds are considered safe for children. Sometimes a desperate medical doctor will use a drug to help a child. The reluctance is because these meds can have troubling effects on kids—or, in some cases, the effects (and possible long-term risks) aren't known well enough for doctors to feel comfortable prescribing them to kids.

Drug companies keep records of their medications' effects on children, but they do not recommend drugs for children because of the litigation factor. It is unethical to do double-blind drug studies on children, so the drug companies gather information from psychiatrists who use these untested drugs as a last resort. Some doctors may recommend these drugs in extremely urgent cases. If a child becomes homicidal or suicidal, these drugs may be the only alternative.

Because bipolar disorder is assumed to be genetic and chemical, sometimes the therapist is considered unimportant. Research by the NIMH (National Institute for Mental Health) shows otherwise; psychotherapy is known to be effective in treating bipolar disorder.

Psychotherapy usually has no adverse side effects. Antidepressants, however, are cause for concern. Several recent high-profile studies have linked antidepressants to higher suicide rates in bipolar teens. One way to lessen this risk is to counterbalance an antidepressant by using it in conjunction with a mood stabilizer or other similar drug for bipolar disorder, along with psychotherapy.

Red Flag _____

Bipolar medications are notorious for causing a host of side effects, ranging from weight gain and dizziness to those as serious as suicidal tendencies. Make sure you research all of a drug's possible side effects, and keep alert for signs of adverse reactions. (On the bright side, side effects such as dizziness and fatigue often lessen or disappear completely once the body becomes accustomed to a medication.) Before you get scared off by complicated descriptions of side effects, ask someone whose child has taken the drug. Your best information may come from another parent who has experienced the drug's effects on her child.

Often, a doctor will start treatment with the mildest possible drug, gradually moving up to more powerful (and perhaps riskier) medications if the initial meds don't provide enough improvement. There are also doctors who start with an amount of medication that will be sure to zap the bipolar disorder and then gradually wean the patient to a dosage that allows a better quality of life. Some doctors use the diagnosis to determine the medication. Other doctors assess the "clusters of behavior" and provide medication that will address the clusters.

Many people assume that medication makes a person with BP lethargic. This is not a correct assumption. Many times the patient hasn't slept and has been stressed out for so long that he needs a rest. Once the medication connects the body and brain back together, the patient realizes how exhausted he is. Let him catch up on his rest first, and then decide about the effects of the medication.

Delayed Effects, Dependency, and Withdrawal

Keep a few things in mind when it comes to bipolar meds. First, most of these meds must accumulate in a person's system for a while before they start to work. This is why patients often complain that a medication isn't working after a few days. Generally, you need to wait at least a few weeks to really evaluate a drug's results.

Almost all bipolar medications are non-addictive. Some sleep medications used with bipolar disorder may be addictive. As with any sleep medication, some medications carry the risk of dependency. Discuss this with your child's doctor. If substance abuse is a concern, your child may also need a drug and alcohol counselor. Doctors are not usually trained in addiction and may not know that an addictive drug can trigger other addictions.

Additionally, some BP meds can cause serious withdrawal (and, in some cases, major negative side effects) if they are stopped suddenly. For that reason, a doctor will usually dictate a plan in which the patient gradually lessens his dosage over several weeks, to avoid an abrupt shock to the system. This is often referred to as the "weaning process."

Advice for Parents

This is all scary stuff, to be sure. So what's a parent to do? The most important thing parents can do is educate themselves as much as possible about bipolar meds, so they can make informed decisions.

Unfortunately, we cannot tell you exactly what to do here. These are individual decisions that parents must make in conjunction with their child's doctors and therapist. If the child is old enough, he or she should be involved in the decision, as well. There are usually no black and white answers, only shades of gray. Pick the lightest shade of gray. One good thing is that any decision you make is likely to be reversible. Mostly, you can see how it goes and change it if it's not working. The previous treatment decisions in the testimonials were all different and based upon the parties involved, the personality of the child, and the treatment available.

> **Mental Note** _____
>
> Some bipolar medications can lose their effectiveness after being taken for a while—or can begin to work differently as a child ages, especially during and after puberty. The child and his parents need to monitor any changes in the medication's effects and report this information to the doctor promptly.

Parents need to ask themselves these questions when contemplating medication options:

- ◆ Have I researched the medications enough to feel comfortable discussing them?

- ◆ Am I (and my child) prepared to handle possible side effects?

- ◆ If my child's symptoms aren't severe, would I be more comfortable starting off with a mild medication?

- ◆ Is my child mature and responsible enough to take his medication on his own?

And here are some questions to ask your child's doctor:

- ◆ Are there side effects I need to be aware of?

- ◆ Will this drug interact negatively with any other medications, prescription or over-the-counter (OTC)?

- ◆ If my child has other medical problems, will this medication cause any complications?

- ◆ If we decide to discontinue use of this drug, is there a weaning process involved?

- ◆ What can I do to adjunct the medication (omega-3, having a routine, psychotherapy, etc.)?

School Problems

School can be a challenging and stressful place for any kid, but it can be especially tough for young people with bipolar disorder. Kids whose symptoms are severe or not well-controlled may have serious difficulties socializing with other kids due to depression, social anxiety, tendencies toward isolation, or manic phases. At times their emotions may be magnified.

These kids are much more likely to have behavior problems, act out, or defy authority—which can make them unpopular with classmates and teachers alike. Even kids who are on a good medication regimen may not be in the clear. The side effects of their meds may cause them problems in school, making them tired in the mornings, for example.

If the child's school staff is cooperative and willing to help accommodate his special needs, that can make a huge difference. Parents should keep the child's school well-informed and make sure the channels of communication are open, allowing the school personnel to best handle the child's particular needs.

An online chat room for bipolar kids can suffice for your child to talk anonymously with other bipolar kids about school, medication, and so on. They're much more likely to share inner feelings if it's anonymous.

Therapy and counseling can also go a long way in helping a child fit in better at school and deal with any problems that may arise.

The Least You Need to Know

◆ BP can be more difficult to diagnose and treat in young people.

◆ Symptoms can change or worsen as a child ages, especially around the time of puberty.

◆ Many BP drugs are recommended only for adults because of their negative or unknown effects on kids. Side effects can range from mild to severe, although some are only temporary.

◆ Check out websites for the newest information on bipolar kids from time to time. You may also find some online bipolar kids chat rooms.

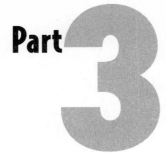

Part 3

Treatment

For someone with bipolar disorder, getting treatment (and, more important, the right kind of treatment) can literally be a lifesaver. In this part,
we'll cover the various treatment options available, including medication,
therapy, and—when necessary—hospitalization. We'll also show you how to
formulate a treatment plan.

Organizing a Treatment Plan

In This Chapter

- ◆ The six "-ates" method
- ◆ What's right for you?
- ◆ The difference between happy and "too happy"

Living with bipolar disorder can be a challenge in many ways. Just planning and managing your treatment can be daunting. In this chapter, we'll help you figure out how to organize your treatment plan so it's easier to handle.

The Importance of a Treatment Plan

Before we get into tips for organizing a treatment plan, we should explain why you need one. Although some people with bipolar disorder think (at least at first) that they can wing it, by handling each symptom or problem as it arises, that's just asking for trouble.

For one thing, as we've already mentioned, many signs of trouble (such as a manic episode) aren't obvious until they are already in full swing. At that point, you'd be forced to scramble to do damage control, and you may not be able to or even want to. It's much better to have a plan in place to treat—or even better, prevent—the situation. After a manic episode, your lobe may go off-line for a couple months, taking your executive functions with it. It's pretty hard to organize and prioritize with your lobe off-line and no access to executive functions.

Also treatments such as medications can take a while to start working. You need to be proactive and have a plan in place—and in progress—before you reach a crisis point.

Plus, managing bipolar disorder involves numerous different tasks (daily medications, therapy, lifestyle issues), so having everything put together in an organized plan will make your life much easier.

When to Enact a Treatment Plan

How about now? A well-organized treatment plan should consist of long-term solutions for managing your life with bipolar disorder. By creating a plan, you're saying, "Bipolar disorder will not run or ruin my life. I will learn how to deal with my disorder as part of my life."

Most effective treatment plans include a trusted friend or family member; psychotherapy with a mental health professional; medication prescribed by a doctor; and lifestyle changes such as a healthful diet, regular sleep, and regular exercise. Timing is everything when organizing a treatment plan, and the time is now. Ever try to go on a diet tomorrow? There are *so* many tomorrows. What better time to organize a treatment plan than while you are reading this book, eh? Go get a paper, pencil, and highlighter—we'll wait for you.

No, really, get it now!

Good. Now, take notes.

For someone in an acute phase of BP, such as a manic episode, the only viable treatment may be hospitalization. The goal of treatment during any acute episode is simply to end the episode. Write that down on your treatment program as a last resort. However, you can create a treatment plan and successfully put it into action between acute episodes or during times of relative normalcy. The goal is to prevent the frequency of future episodes and reduce the severity of episodic symptoms when they do occur.

With a well-organized treatment plan, nearly everyone with bipolar disorder can experience substantial relief from their symptoms. Stability in one's life is key to achieving stability in one's mood. Therefore, bipolar people must establish healthy habits in every area their lives to encourage long-term mood stability. This approach to life is elementary, and applicable to anyone regardless of his or her mental health status. However, it may be more important for bipolar people—and may be more difficult for them to commit to. For example, many people can successfully alternate between a day shift work schedule and night shift schedule, but for someone with bipolar disorder, this kind of erratic sleep schedule can trigger an acute phase of mania or psychosis.

The Six "-ates"

To make things easy, we've boiled down your treatment plan into six tasks which we like to call the six "-ates" (because they each end in "-ate").

Separate

Many people with BP become emotionally dependent upon a spouse or significant other. The bipolar tendency toward impulsivity combined with an eternal search for activities that make them feel better make falling in love exciting and dangerous.

Mental Note _____

We suggest you complete the six tasks in the order they are given here, but ultimately it is your decision to do them in the order best for you.

New romances promote euphoric feelings, and we may rush into them without much forethought. As a result, relationships can be rocky and sometimes unhealthy for people with BP. It is difficult for them to sever ties with someone they were once intimate with because they experience deeper than normal despair. The loss may trigger an extended depressive episode capable of spoiling every other area of a bipolar person's life. For someone with bipolar disorder, losing a mate can also mean losing a job, due to temporarily losing his or her mind.

That's why many bipolar people remain in verbally and physically abusive relationships that worsen their already troubled mental conditions. The intense pain of a quick detachment can be so terrifying that they prolong their long-term suffering by maintaining bad relationships.

If you know your mate causes you undue stress and has triggered mood episodes in the past, you should get the advice of someone you trust and possibly separate from your partner while you organize your treatment plan. You can tell your mate you are going to stay with a friend for a time to clear your head and work some things out. If you cannot separate yourself from a mate who has a negative impact on your bipolar disorder, be sure to make that issue a priority in individual therapy. You may have children or know that separating will trigger your mate into making things worse. If so, keeping the peace while you work out your treatment plan may be your best option.

Once you eliminate or reduce contact with persons who stress and upset you, the next step is to reach out to someone you can trust.

Delegate

Appoint a person you trust to help you formulate and institute your treatment plan. The person should be someone you already call upon when you need help or support, someone who has expressed concern or told you that you need to make some changes. If you don't trust anyone close to you, you may find someone at local support meetings to buddy up with.

The appointed person must understand what you intend to do and agree to help you do it. Explain that you believe you may need treatment and that you intend to seek a mental assessment from a doctor. You may want to ask the person to come to the doctor with you.

It is very important to be in a safe and understanding environment when you begin trying medications and other types of therapies, in case you suffer side effects like nausea or insomnia. You may ask to stay with this person for a few weeks. You can also stay at hotels or shelters nearby if your friend cannot accommodate your request. If you're lucky enough to have nearby friends or family, you can get them all together and ask for assistance. Stay a few days with one and a few with another in turn or rotation.

Sometimes this is difficult for one appointee to handle, so you may involve several people instead. Approach your loved ones with the help of one trusted friend, to make breaking the news about your situation and your plan of action less difficult.

Another important consideration is damage control. (Before you approach your circle of friends and family, be sure to read Chapter 20.)

Mending personal and professional relationships that have become collateral damage of untreated bipolar disorder is difficult. Apologies need to be made and explanations are deserved. Just as you are a victim of bipolar disorder, so, too, are the people in your world.

Educate

It's important for you to educate yourself about your condition. Talk therapy or cognitive therapy actually creates new neural pathways over time. Examining your life history with a professional (such as a counselor) can result in major behavioral changes. You can literally learn how to "feel" differently about yourself, the world, and your place in it.

In order to change your feelings, however, you need to understand what has happened to you, what you have done in response, and why. Therapists aren't psychics; they are trained to ask the right questions and help you to find and understand your own answers. If the therapist is the right one for you, you will leave a session saying, "I did not know that about myself." You may have an epiphany or a moment of realization that will bring about positive, permanent change.

Therapy sessions can often be extremely emotional, bordering on traumatic. Reliving unpleasant experiences in a therapy session will help you resolve or heal the emotional issues that complicate your bipolar illness. It will help you understand the relationship between the features of your mental illness and features of your environment.

Keep journals of what you learn in therapy to review after the session, when you are less emotional. Keep track of your mood cycles on a calendar and try to identify what triggered each individual episode. Learn what substances or activities you need to avoid by recording daily events. Take what you learn and share it with your appointee or your circle of trusted helpers to reinforce in your own mind what you learn and to educate them about your problems. The more they understand your problems, the better able they will be to help you get well.

Medicate

When we say medicate, we mean with prescribed drugs—not illicit drugs. Once you have chosen the right mental health professional, you and she will choose a medication or medications to modify the operation of your neurotransmitters.

Everyone reacts to medication differently, so remember that finding the right medication may require some trial and error. Mood episodes are recurring problems. Bipolar disorder is almost always a lifelong affliction. Most experts suggest thinking of your illness as similar to diabetes or asthma. You will need to treat it every day for as long as you live. Don't stop taking your medication or switch to another without first informing your doctor! Some bipolar patients are lucky, achieving therapeutic effects from the first medications they try (albeit after a period of side effects). Others are not so fortunate and must go through a process of trial and error before finding the appropriate medication.

It is very important to eliminate illicit drugs and alcohol when you begin your prescription regimen. For instance, using alcohol will intensify many undesirable side effects and block the therapeutic value of many psychoactive drugs. It will become difficult or impossible to know how effective your prescriptions are if you self-medicate during this important medical process.

Motivate

You can keep yourself motivated by trying new activities. Even low-impact exercise like taking a walk around your neighborhood can make a big difference in maintaining your mood stability. Movement is imperative to mental and physical health because it boosts endorphins and serotonin levels. Yoga, aerobics, and tennis are examples of activities (depending on your fitness level) to start with a day. Then build up to three days a week as you become more fit. Extend your exercise by 15 minutes, play one extra game, or walk one extra block.

Switch it up: you don't have to always do the same exercises. Different activities use different muscles. So you might try yoga one week. The next week, try three days of jogging and four days of yoga. The weeks after that, try swimming or cycling. Be careful that you don't manically exercise. Set limits on the time you will spend exercising once you get into the swing of it.

Your brain really is like a muscle, and it can grow and become fit when it is stimulated. Puzzles and books on new interesting topics are great for your brain's fitness, but so is putting the rest of your body in motion. Drinking alcohol, on the other hand, kills neurons and over time will reduce the size of your brain and limit its functions. Taking lithium or antidepressants has been shown in numerous studies to increase the number and function of neurons and glial cells, thus increasing brain size and function. Be sure to go out, get some fresh air, move your body, and smell the roses. A fit brain is a healthy one!

As an added benefit to people with BP (about time!), it has recently been discovered that lithium and other medications used to treat BP actually prevent Alzheimer's disease.

> **Research Says**
>
> Brain studies of dancers show that learning and practicing new dances strengthens the brain's motor areas and cognitive areas. Learning and executing the new movements actually facilitates the growth of new neurons. It enables you to set your mind in motion, rather than letting your mind wander around in an undirected way.

Meditate

Find a healthy balance between times of activity and rest. Rest, relaxation, and sleep are essential for a healthy brain. While you sleep, your brain reorganizes information that will be used when you are awake. It dissects and analyzes problems and then constructs solutions to the situations that you encounter. The old advice to "sleep on it" is truly a sensible way to make sound decisions.

Even if you just lie in bed quietly and meditate on your day with your eyes closed, your brain benefits from receiving far less input than usual and thereby gets to rest. This is one reason not to get upset or frustrated when you can't sleep. Even if you just lie in bed awake with your eyes closed and meditate, you are still benefiting from a sleeplike state. You are also more likely to eventually fall asleep because you are relaxed and not stressing yourself over being awake. Allowing your thoughts to drift freely or allowing yourself to concentrate on the slow rhythms of breathing will serve as relaxation therapies that will keep your body and brain fresh and rejuvenated. Meditation actually gets you into your prefrontal lobe, after which you can usually see the bigger picture a bit better.

You may want to take a formal course in transcendental meditation. There has been much research done on this technique and, as they say, it's all good. Transcendental meditation is not a religion. For those who are religious, prayer is a great form of meditation. There are also some good books on meditation. Ask your librarian which ones people find most useful.

Consistency is paramount to your treatment plan's success. Your level of commitment to the plan you invent will be directly proportionate to the level of relief and mood stability you will enjoy. So stick to it. Initially it may be hard to institute these new routines in your life, but keep at it and it will become effortless.

Planning Your Diet

Food is medicine. Therefore, meal planning is an important part of your treatment plan. Brains function best with a steady, reliable stream of quality nutrients. It's a good idea to devote some time one day a week to prepare healthy meals for the week. If you shop and prepare foods ahead of time, you are less likely to eat food that is bad for you.

You should have three meals spaced throughout the day and wholesome snacks in between to get you through the day. Diet is intertwined with medicine. They both go into your mouth and are digested and used by your body. They both create physiological changes that may be good or bad. The mood and food connection has been recognized for centuries and is an integral part of general well-being, no matter who you are.

American diets are often riddled with tasty treats that lack any nutritional value. It seems strange, but many Americans are both overfed and malnourished. They aren't eating the right foods to gain essential nutrients. Eating plenty of fruits and vegetables will provide the necessary vitamins and minerals for your body to maintain its optimal health. Vitamins and supplement pills are just that—supplements, not replacements. To be well nourished, you need to eat a variety of foods. Your body needs over 40 known nutrients to keep fit, and no single food can supply all of them.

Eating right is a must for everyone, but people with bipolar disorder should eat more of some foods and stay away from others.

Red Flag

Many of the medications prescribed to treat bipolar disorder can rob the body of vitamins and minerals. Your body uses up B vitamins, for instance, when it breaks down certain antidepressants.

Natural food stores usually have a liquid vitamin B_{12} that you take under the tongue. It tastes pretty good, too! Making sure you have the vitamins necessary to process your medication and carry out all your normal physical activities is a must. You should take a high-quality multivitamin daily in addition to your well-balanced diet.

Many of the medications used to stabilize mood can promote weight gain. This is why you should avoid alcohol and sugar. Foods made with simple sugars or carbohydrates provide little nourishment but plenty of calories. Sugar is often listed on labels under names most people don't recognize. Start reading food labels and avoid those products containing corn syrup or fructose, maltose, dextrose, sucrose, fructose, lactose, or polydextrose. The "oses" lead to grosses. Sugar is metabolized and stored as fat. Alcohol is metabolized into sugar which is then stored as fat. Alcohol is a big problem for your liver, which may be busy breaking down your medications. As mentioned previously, mixing medication and alcohol can also cause bipolar symptoms to worsen.

The omega-3 fatty acids docosahexaenoic acid (DHA) and eicosapentaenoic acid (EPA) are essential nutrients for good health, but they are particularly important for bipolar disorder as preventatives and to smooth out those peaks and valleys you get even on medication. DHA plays a direct role in brain development and lifetime maintenance, whereas EPA is influential in maintaining mood stability. DHA and EPA generate neuroprotective metabolites (byproducts). Fish oil DHA/EPA triglycerides supplements come in pill form, are found in most drug stores, and are reasonably priced. When taken with meals there is rarely a burp, so you almost never have to taste the fishiness of the oil. One psychiatrist recommends 2,000 mg of omega-3 a day for maintenance and 7,500 to 11,000 mg a day when unstable.

As always, discuss your diet plan with your doctor to make sure you are getting everything you need and in appropriate amounts.

Mental Note _____

If you put omega-3 capsules in the freezer overnight and take them the next morning frozen, you are unlikely to get the burps.

Doing What's Right for You

Sometimes you may have to leave it up to others to determine what is right for you. If you are mentally incapable of making good decisions, then the right thing to do is to select people you can trust to help you make decisions until you are well enough to make them for yourself. In a 12-step program, this is the "surrender" step. Surrender does not mean "give up." It means that you do what you can and as much as is appropriate, then you leave it up to a higher power. The higher power could be someone you trust whose prefrontal lobe is functioning better than yours for the time being.

When you are operating at maximum brain function, you have to decide what is best for you, making provisions in case you become temporarily incapacitated. This is when you appoint someone to be your overseer if you slip on the banana peel and implement preventative strategies so you don't slip. Don't become overconfident just because you feel fine today. Life has a way of throwing banana peels in your path. Plan for it, and if it doesn't happen, great. It won't hurt to have a plan, and it may save your life as you know it.

If you are experiencing ego, arrogance, and entitlement, it is not the time to plan or make big decisions. If you feel "too good," it is time to call your doctor. There is a difference between being happy and being high. If you look hard, you will see the difference. Most people with BP know what this means. People with BP have experienced being "too happy" and know the difference between that racing feeling and being content and peaceful. Happiness is a big-picture phenomenon. "Too happy" is fleeting.

Bumps in the Road to Well-Being

Do not be discouraged if your initial attempts at any of these steps fail. The people around you may not understand BP and may react badly to your plan to seek psychiatric evaluation.

Parents

Parents are especially prone to negativity when first told of your intentions. Parents often feel as though they are to blame if you are suffering from a mental illness, that they must have done a poor job of raising you and are responsible for any mental defect you have developed. They may feel embarrassed and to blame for having passed on defective traits to their offspring and not want their "weaknesses" to become a diagnosed reality—or, worse, a public scandal.

> **Mental Note**
>
> Proof that mental illness is widespread, recognizable, and treatable can help relieve parents of some shock, guilt, and dismay. A list of symptoms provided by a well-respected national organization might help them to accept your diagnosis and reconsider their contrary positions.

If you make your case to them quietly and clearly, and then remain calm if they argue that you don't need a psychiatrist, they will be more likely to accept your plans. You should explain that you are sorry they feel the way they do, but that seeking help is what you believe you need to do. Leaving them some literature to stumble upon the next day is often a good idea. It shows you have done your homework and that your beliefs are founded on legitimate information. A fact sheet printed out from the National Institutes of Mental Health (NIMH) website could enlighten them to how many people suffer from mental illnesses and from bipolar disorder in particular.

Spouses

Spouses may wrongly believe that you can just try harder to work out your problems and that seeking professional help will not solve anything. If your spouse doesn't support your decision to get help, a number of common fears may be to blame. He may fear that once you have help you may be less emotionally dependent on him—and that you may ultimately leave him. Spouses often worry that they themselves have created the problem from which you seek relief.

Some spouses fear that psychiatry will be expensive. They feel embarrassed by the prospect of word getting out to friends and neighbors. Like your parents, they feel you are a reflection of them. If you are mentally ill, what are they by association? It may help to tell them that bipolar is considered a physiological rather than a psychiatric illness by a number of renowned psychiatrists (roundtable in May 2008, medscape. com).

Most spouses worth the title will agree without too much convincing that you should give mental help a try if you feel you need it. You should explain that the happier and more stable you are, the happier and more stable your relationship will be. This should make perfect sense to your spouse if he has tried to help you during a bout of depression and failed. It will also make sense to him if your illness has caused you to treat him poorly in the past.

Older Children

Adult children are another group who may resist the reality of your mental illness and your need for mental help. Teenagers are especially touchy about matters of public opinion. You may opt to wait until you have been diagnosed and stabilized before you explore the topic with children who are young adults. Once you are satisfied that your diagnosis is correct and that various therapies are working for you, you may want to tell your children that they are also at risk of developing an inherited illness.

Taking your children along to a support meeting or individual therapy session is an excellent way to help them understand your situation. Your therapist may be better at helping them understand the role they can play in your treatment plan. For example, a child may become your exercise partner and encourage you to be active. Or an older child may be able to drive you on errands while you adjust to new medications that say "Do not drive" on the bottle.

Involving your children in your treatment plan promotes the understanding necessary to mend damage to your relationship attributable to your mood episodes. If your relationship with your children and your spouse is substantially strained by your past behavior, then family counseling may be an ideal solution.

Research Says

Early detection and treatment have been shown to dramatically change disease progression in favor of the patient. Having your children evaluated by a mental health professional at any age is appropriate, but it is especially important when mental illness exists among previous generations.

Employers

Research indicates that as many as one in five American workers suffers from a mental illness. The government protects these workers from discrimination under the Americans with Disabilities Act. According to the act, you cannot be fired because you have a mental illness. However, you can be fired for missing too many days of work if you do not provide the necessary evidence of disability at the appropriate time.

You are not under any obligation to inform your employer that you are mentally ill, but not doing so can work to your disadvantage if you do require accommodation. If you choose to inform your employer, be sure to speak with him privately.

Mental Note

The law prevents your employer from sharing any disability you disclose to him in private with anyone else in your workplace.

Most people don't know how to deal with mental illness because they don't know very much about it. You can be vague about your problem if you prefer and use a generic terms like "brain disorder" or "neurological illness." If you want to reveal your actual diagnosis, be sure to have a brochure or pamphlet that will provide basic information on hand. Your employer probably will not want to hear a long explanation of your biochemical imbalance or your life history. Assure him that you are still able to do your job and that your productivity will remain satisfactory. Explain that you may need to leave work early for a therapy appointment or make up work on a weekend if a new medication disagrees with you.

Tell your employer that you will notify him in advance as much as possible if you must miss work due to your illness and that you will provide documentation from your doctor for your absence. Many employers will allow you to work from home if you don't feel able to come to the office. As long as your employer hears that you have a plan and that you will be able to manage your condition, he will most likely cooperate with you fully.

If your employer treats you unfairly after being informed of your illness, you should contact legal services for your protection.

The Importance of Sharing

Letting friends, family, and employers in on your illness is a daunting task to say the least. You should keep a few things about disclosure in mind. First, you are paving the way to a more tolerant and understanding world for other mentally ill people.

Life with mental illness is hard enough without being forced to endure prejudices and humiliations. Every person who truly likes and respects you who learns that you are mentally ill will still like and respect you. They will carry the understanding and good-will they have toward you and apply it in dealings with other sufferers. Like the brave people who spoke out in the civil rights era, you are a social pioneer! If you come out of the bipolar closet and promote public awareness about mental illness, you do all of us a great service.

By doing what is right for you and informing others, you are helping to take away the stigma surrounding mental illness. Keep in mind, there is a stigma. It is an unfortunate reality. You may prefer to divulge as little information as possible instead of becoming an advocate for mental illness de-stigma.

The Least You Need to Know

- If you implement and follow the six "-ates" system for your contextual (big picture) treatment plan, the process will be much easier.

- Being "too happy" requires a call to your doctor and the recognition that no long-term decisions should be made about your life.

- It's a good idea to select a trusted friend or professional for those times you are not functioning at 100 percent.

- Medication exists to help manage your BP. It may not make everything all right, and it may require a period of adjustment and experimentation before it is the most helpful.

- Have your treatment plan lined up before you slip on the banana peel. Not that you are planning to slip, but if you do, having a plan is like insurance.

11

Medications

In This Chapter

♦ Information from the National Institute of Mental Health (NIMH)

♦ Phenomenological feedback from health-care professionals on the effects of medication

♦ Medication-related dangers to keep in mind

♦ The most reliable medication options

Medication plays a critical role in a treatment plan for a patient with bipolar disorder. When prescribed and taken properly, medication can be a lifesaver, literally. But there are also issues related to bipolar medications, which can involve significant side effects for some, and other concerns.

In this chapter, we describe the different types of medications prescribed for BP and explain the pros and cons related to them.

An Important Disclaimer

This chapter is based upon recommendations by the National Institute of Mental Health (NIMH) and phenomenological feedback (observations) from mental health professionals, including people dealing with bipolar disorder in the trenches every day (psychologists, social workers, counselors, psychiatrists, medical doctors, nurse practitioners, nurses, and other medical professionals).

The author of this chapter has studied psychotropic medication, is certified in psychoactive substance abuse disorders, worked with medical doctors for 10 years, is a psychologist, and has done more than 6,000 psychological evaluations—but is not a medical doctor.

This chapter is not intended to substitute for supervision, consultation, or expert advice regarding mental health assessment or treatment for specific cases or specific individuals. This material is for educational purposes only. The information in this chapter is presented as accurately and competently as possible with the opinions and observations of health-care professionals and the NIMH. This information may change as new discoveries are made. Always check with your physician before assuming accuracy. The nice thing about the NIMH is that they have a website and it gets updated. Even if this book becomes old, you can still find the newest information on their website. NIMH is funded by the government, so access is granted to everyone and there is no copyright.

Medication Basics

First of all, medication does not necessarily make everything okay. If you're lucky, it might. For many people with bipolar disorder, medication makes the bipolar disorder more manageable. Many times I have heard someone say to a person with bipolar disorder, "If you just took your medication, everything would be okay." It's not that simple.

For most people, bipolar medication stabilizes bipolar disorder so it can be managed. But it can be difficult to find the right medication. If you give up before finding the medication that works for you, the alternative is bipolar symptoms that can ruin your entire life (by making you gamble away your life savings, lose all your friends, contract a sexually transmitted disease, or feel like jumping off the Golden Gate Bridge). However, more discoveries are being made. If we had a few more brilliant scientists looking into bipolar disorder, I bet we would have better treatment, better medications, and a better understanding of bipolar disorder.

Traditional Medications

Quite a few different medications (and types of medications) are used to treat bipolar disorder. Let's start by discussing the traditional ones.

Lithium

For many years, lithium was the main medication prescribed for bipolar disorder. It was the first FDA-approved mood stabilization medication, and many doctors still consider it the best.

The drug companies are always coming out with new medications (as well they should), and of course they advertise and promote the newer drugs. When is the last time you saw a television advertisement for lithium? The companies don't need to advertise it and the patent has expired, so lithium is not as lucrative as the newer, patented drugs.

I am not criticizing the drug companies; their role is to find new medications, fund research, and market their products. It is the role of the medical community to treat the disorder with the best resources available without prejudice or preferential treatment to drug companies.

Almost no current medications that I know of are perfect for bipolar disorder. If you want "natural," lithium is perhaps the most natural you can get in a prescription drug. I have met many people who have taken lithium religiously for 25 or 35 years, and I have not seen any bipolar kindling effect (getting worse from lack of treatment). Most people I know who have taken lithium every day are alive and well. They have not jumped off the Golden Gate Bridge. They have raised children and are still around for their grandchildren.

I am not selling lithium. It may not work for you. The first couple months of treatment can be challenging, with the drug causing the shakes, weight gain, and other side effects. For most people, the effects improve and they learn to live with and compensate for them. Make sure your doctor takes regular blood levels to check for therapeutic levels and lithium toxicity. Learn the symptoms of lithium toxicity so that you can alert your

 Red Flag

A patient may have to switch to another medication after decades of taking lithium. Lithium is a salt, and salts affect the kidneys. Years and years of taking lithium can cause the kidneys to get worn out, so the patient must switch to a medication that does not metabolize in the kidneys.

doctor if you experience them. Ask a relative or spouse to be aware of the signs and to remind you to take your medication.

The good news is that you can't drink when you are taking lithium. The bad news is that you can't drink when you are taking lithium. Some doctors may allow their patients an occasional glass of wine, but check with your doctor. You won't need to self-medicate with alcohol while you are on lithium, anyway.

The phenomenological reports (observations) that this author has received suggest that lithium is good for preventing mania, but that its antidepressant qualities take a while to work.

The NIMH is studying lithium (see NIMH –15 on their website), as it may block development of Alzheimer's disease by significantly reducing the production of beta amyloid, which causes cell death in Alzheimer's. Nonsteroidal anti-inflammatory drugs (NSAIDs) behave like lithium in this regard, but with a slightly different mechanism. Lithium levels should be monitored when you initiate or discontinue use of NSAIDs (which include ibuprofen, naprosyn, and indomethacin). Research shows that the NSAIDs block excretion of lithium through the kidneys and therefore increase lithium levels. Research is still pending on whether NSAIDs, which operate by a mechanism similar to that of lithium, can effectively be used to treat bipolar disorder. The research is almost complete and it looks like the anti-inflammatories do show efficacy for bipolar disorder.

Anticonvulsant Medications

Some medications that are primarily designed as anticonvulsants have also proven effective in treating mania. Valproate was FDA-approved in 1995 for treatment of mania and is often used in combination with lithium. Other anticonvulsant meds are being studied to determine how well they work in stabilizing mood cycles.

Carbamazepine is an older drug used to treat bipolar disorder as well as seizures. It is also used for impulse control disorders.

Lamotrigine has been approved by the FDA for bipolar disorder and it is a good preventative for episodes. The dosage is usually low with minimal weight gain or sexual side effects. It is usually titrated up slowly so the patient avoids the Stevens-Johnson rash, which is rare, but can be serious. People have reported that this medication makes them feel normal. People who are very functional seem to do well on this medication. Others with more severe bipolar disorder may need an augmentation to this drug. This is a preventative drug, and the only drug considered preventative by many medical professionals.

Although psychiatrists have traditionally been responsible for prescribing bipolar meds, primary care physicians are beginning to prescribe BP medications more often and may be the starting point for people with BP more in the future. In severe cases, people with bipolar disorder should see a psychiatrist for treatment, but a family physician may be able to prescribe something to reduce symptoms until the patient can see a psychiatrist.

Mood Stabilizers

Mood stabilizers are usually prescribed to help control bipolar disorder. Several different types of mood stabilizers are available. In general, people with bipolar disorder continue treatment with mood stabilizers for long periods of time. Other medications are added when necessary for shorter periods, to treat episodes of mania or depression that emerges.

Many mood-stabilizing medications are not recommended for children, because their long-term effects are unknown and because they might pose a risk to the developing bodies of younger patients.

Women with bipolar disorder who become pregnant should consult with a doctor as soon as possible to learn how to deal with their medications. Some medication can have a harmful effect on the fetus. See Chapter 18 for more information.

Antidepressants

Tricyclic antidepressants and SSRIs can trigger manic episodes in people with bipolar disorder. These drugs show no efficacy for bipolar depression anyway. People being treated for unipolar depression with a tricyclic or SSRI may find out they are actually bipolar when the drug triggers an episode.

If bipolar disorder runs in the family, the doctor may want to protect people with a possible undiagnosed bipolar disorder from a bipolar episode with lithium, valproate, or other bipolar medication.

Atypicals

Atypical drugs are second-generation drugs that work differently than the first-generation antipsychotics (Haldol, Thorozine, and so on). Most of the atypicals work on serotonin receptors and dopamine receptors. Researchers are currently studying atypical antipsychotic medications (such as risperidone, clozapine, and olanzapine) to evaluate their potential for treating bipolar disorder. Some atypicals have been approved by the FDA for bipolar disorder through successful double-blind studies. Some of these meds are helpful in treating mania or depression.

The following are examples of atypical drugs:

- Clozapine
- Risperidone
- Olanzapine
- Quetiapine
- Ziprasidone
- Aripiprazole
- Paliperidone
- Asenapine
- Iloperidone
- Melperone (approved in Europe; clinical trial in the United States)

The FDA approved risperidone for the short-term treatment of the mixed and manic states associated with bipolar disorder and for the treatment of irritability in children.

Olanzapine is approved by the FDA for bipolar mania and as a maintenance medication for same. Olanzapine is probably one of the best medications for stabilizing bipolar episodes. The biggest side effect is weight gain. It has also been associated with diabetes.

Quetiapine is considered a mood stabilizer and is approved by the FDA to treat both the highs and lows of bipolar disorder. It is used sometimes as an adjunct medication for sleep as well.

Aripiprazole is used to treat the symptoms of bipolar disorder. It is approved by the FDA for bipolar mania. Out of the antipsychotics, you will probably gain the least amount of weight on this medication.

The other drugs listed above are newer and can be found on the Internet. Just because a drug is new does not mean it is better. There is always a certain hype about a new drug until it is used in the public and certain limitations come to light. This author's recommendation is to stick to the drugs that have a history, since we know more about the good, the bad, and the ugly of that particular drug.

Insomnia and Benzodiazepines

You can find help for insomnia with a benzodiazepine medication such as clonazepam, lorazepam, alprazolam, or diazepam. Since these medications may be habit forming, they are best prescribed on a short-term basis. Other types of sedative medications, such as zolpidem, can be used instead, but are not recommended long term. Eszopiclone seems to help people stay asleep as well as get to sleep and is recommended by some for longer term. Since sleep is a major concern for people with bipolar disorder, it is better to take something to help sleep, rather than to not sleep.

Trazedone is non-addicting and is used by many with BP to get to sleep. Diphenhydramine is an over-the-counter antihistamine and is popularly used for sleep. Always check with you doctor to make sure the sleep aids are compatible with your bipolar meds.

Medication Changes

It's fairly common for people with bipolar disorder to need occasional (or even frequent) adjustments to their medication regimen. Your doctor should monitor your overall health—specifically, things like kidney function and liver enzymes—and should make immediate adjustments if you show any signs of adverse effects from your meds. You may also notice that your medication starts to become less effective over time, in which case the dosage may need to be increased or the drug may need to be replaced with a more effective alternative.

Sometimes it is difficult to find a medication that works. You may be lucky and get it right the first time, or you may go through many medications. Don't forget that the medication doesn't make everything okay; it just helps you manage bipolar disorder. For example, a patient who went through many medications, but none seemed to stabilize him. Finally, trifluoperazine did. It is an antipsychotic medication that also treats anxiety. It is used in the treatment of the manic phase of bipolar disorder as well as for non-psychotic anxiety.

Red Flag

While it may be necessary for your doctor to make changes in your medication, you should never do this on your own. Tinkering with your medication routine—or dropping a medication altogether—can cause serious problems.

The Latest Options

Metformin has been shown to prevent diabetes and mitigate weight gain for people with BP taking medications that tend to cause weight gain. The studies are small, but look promising. Metformin is the most popular anti-diabetic drug in the United States and one of the most prescribed drugs.

OCD and bipolar disorder are very difficult to treat when comorbid. The medications for OCD (usually SSRIs) exacerbate bipolar disorder. First, make sure that the obsessions are caused by OCD. OCD obsessions are fear driven. If the obsessions are not fear driven, then they likely are obsessions accompanying bipolar disorder and will reduce with BP medication. Two methods of treatment seem to work if it is truly OCD and bipolar:

◆ Stabilize the patient on a mood stabilizer first. Then introduce the OCD medication.

◆ Olanzapine treatment. Of course, olanzapine may carry a significant weight gain with it.

Trileptal (oxcarbazepine) is a derivative of Tegretol (carbamazepine) and seems to be well liked and well tolerated, based on the positive feedback of many seminar attendees from a total of 16,000. It is purported to have very few side effects and to be effective in treatment.

Private research done in Portland, Maine, showed that thyroid medication seemed to beef up the power of some bipolar meds. The more thyroid medication used, the less bipolar meds needed. The less bipolar meds, the fewer side effects. The thyroid meds usually have no side effects.

Side Effects and Dangers

Unfortunately, many of the medications commonly used to treat bipolar disorder may have some unpleasant side effects, from minor things like dry mouth to more serious stuff like drowsiness, severe anxiety, and extreme dizziness. In some cases, these side effects will lesson or disappear over time. The extreme anxiety or agitation may come from an atypical antipsychotic due to the effect it may have on the serotonin receptors.

Be sure to keep your doctor informed about any side effects you may experience. Any extreme side effects, or anything that might signify an allergic reaction (swelling, especially in the face or throat; vomiting; difficulty breathing; a sudden rash; blurred vision), should be addressed immediately. Call your doctor or go to the ER or your doctor's office right away.

Interactions with Other Meds

It is important that your doctor know about all other medications you are taking. Tell the doctor about over-the-counter medications and natural remedies you may be using. Why? Because an SSRI and the dietary supplement tryptophan can cause serotonin syndrome and make you sick. Why? Because paroxetine and St. John's wort can put you into a coma. Why? Because some medications boost the power of others and some negate the power of others. The safety net built into the system is that your doctor should check all the meds you are on and notice any contraindications. If the doctor doesn't catch one, the pharmacist should. There are also tools on the Internet for you to enter medications and compute the contraindications, if any.

The doctor should also know about any unusual thing you do. If you are a roofer and work on a roof all day, sweating a lot, and you are on lithium, you may need to make some special provisions. First of all, you have to drink a lot of water—which means you have to visit the bathroom more often. If you are on a roof 20 stories high, it isn't convenient to go to the bathroom. The man I am thinking of solved the problem by taking a bucket up on the roof with him.

Sometimes we discover things from the interaction of medications. For example, the thyroid medication boosting the power of bipolar meds discussed earlier. Some interactions are good interactions.

When Meds Make Things Worse

Lithium has been known to make some people feel nauseous and some get the shakes to some degree for the first month. One man vomited 43 times (he counted because he also had OCD). He lost 15 pounds the first week. His psychiatrist had told him to give it some time. Well, lithium just didn't work for him.

Always keep your doctor informed. Your doctor may be able to help and, if the medication just isn't working, will be able to tell you how to come off the medication.

Lamotrigine is an excellent medication for some people. It can put some people's BP into remission. These people take the meds and get no side effects and no symptoms. But one woman who was stabilized on meds after an episode was given lamotrigine to try. Her therapist noticed a rash on her chest and called the doctor.

Unfortunately, she was one of the rare people who get Stevens-Johnson rash, which can be a nasty rash. She couldn't take lamotrigine and the doctor took her off it immediately.

Dangers of Self-Medication

Unfortunately, many people with bipolar disorder "experiment" with their medication. This is a form of self-medication. You are taking the medication regimen out of the hands of your doctor and modifying it to your own agenda. It is okay to adjust your medication, but only with the permission of your doctor. Some doctors will give a range of a certain medication you take and that can be very beneficial to someone who is responsible enough to do it correctly.

If you are reducing your meds to get that "energy," then you are trying to get high off your own mania. You may have an addiction problem that should be addressed by a drug and alcohol counselor.

If you are adjusting your medication right from the get-go, then you are one of those people who think you always know better and you have a poor chance of stabilizing your bipolar disorder.

If you add meds to your regimen without telling the doctor (like that Percocet you saved from your last injury, or that Vicodin you took from your mom's pharmacy), then you need to come clean before you mess up your treatment.

The Least You Need to Know

- ◆ The information in this chapter is for educational purposes only and isn't a substitute for medical advice.

- ◆ Almost all of the bipolar medications come with side effects, although many of them lessen over time.

- ◆ To avoid any negative interactions, it's important to tell your doctor about any medications, over-the-counter drugs, or other substances you are taking.

- ◆ Millions of people are on bipolar medication, enabling them to live a much higher quality of life even with the side effects of their medication.

Chapter 12

Therapy

In This Chapter

◆ Evaluating the available therapy options

◆ Evidence-based therapies

◆ Considering natural therapies

In the previous chapter, we discussed medications used to treat bipolar disorder. While medication is an important part of a BP treatment plan, it is only half of the equation. Most experts believe that a treatment plan combining medication with therapy offers the best chance of success. In this chapter, we'll discuss the benefits of therapy and compare the different types available.

Why Therapy Is Important

You may be thinking, "Okay, I'm taking my meds as directed, and I seem to be doing fine. Why do I need therapy?" Well, you need therapy so you can *keep* doing fine. As you probably already know, manic and depressive episodes are often triggered by stress, emotional distress, relationship troubles, and other situations. If you don't know how to prevent or handle these triggers, you're much more likely to run into trouble.

Therapy can help you recognize your particular triggers and figure out how to deal with them. In addition, therapy can help you identify and resolve hidden issues or traumas that may be buried in your subconscious—past events that may be triggering episodes without you even realizing it.

To sum it up: medication can only do so much. Therapy helps put you in the healthiest possible mental and emotional state, so the medication can do its job with the best results.

If You Are Reluctant to Try Therapy

Lots of people (whether they have BP or not) don't like the idea of therapy. They may be hesitant to try therapy for a variety of reasons. Often, they have misconceptions about what will happen during therapy. They may be uncomfortable with the thought of revealing their innermost feelings and fears to a stranger. Or maybe they simply feel that therapy is just a waste of time (and money).

If you're opposed to the idea of therapy, you need to examine your reasons. We're not saying your reasons aren't valid or logical. Take the fear of revealing your private thoughts. That definitely is a scary thing, and it's only natural to be a bit uncomfortable with the idea. It may help you to know that therapists are trained to be non-judgmental and noncritical. They won't make fun of you or laugh at your problems. They're there to help—and they can't do that unless you open up and let them help you figure out what's troubling you. And you probably already know this, but therapists are required to keep everything you tell them confidential.

The best way to conquer your fear of therapy? Do your research. Talk to friends and relatives who see a therapist and ask them to share feedback or advice. Be warned: not everyone will have had a totally positive experience. Not everyone is a fan of therapy, and some people will have negative things to say about it. Don't totally discount their input, but don't let it sway you too strongly either. Really, the only way to know how you will benefit from therapy is to try it for yourself.

Types of Therapy

Therapy is very personal and individual. No single approach will work best for everyone. Finding the style of therapy that's the best fit for you will give you the best odds of success.

Fortunately, there are quite a few different types of therapy, so you're sure to find at least one that can meet your needs.

No matter what kind of therapist you select, make sure she has education and training in bipolar disorder. Each type of therapist has training in some specialty (or specialties).

A psychologist has a Ph.D., a Psy.D., or an Ed.D. This person is highly trained in the scientific method and usually has one year of internship after the doctoral degree. The

Mental Note

Sometimes because of insurance requirements or limited availability, your psychiatrist may only be able to take care of your medications, so you will need a separate therapist. Your psychiatrist can usually recommend someone who will work with her in a team approach.

Ph.D. is more research oriented, the Psy.D. is more professionally oriented (toward counseling), and the Ed.D. is more learning oriented. In any case, the psychologist takes a psychological approach to the well-being of the patient. A psychologist is licensed by the state.

A psychiatrist is a medical doctor who attended medical school and went on to specialize in psychiatry. These doctors may be schooled in psychoanalysis, but will primarily take a medical approach to the wellness of the patient. They are licensed by the state as psychiatrists.

Counselors come in several types:

◆ A drug and alcohol (D&A) counselor is experienced in counseling people who have substance abuse problems. This person may be a certified addictions counselor and licensed by the state.

◆ A licensed professional counselor (L.P.C.) has a Master's degree and is trained in one or more types of psychotherapy. This therapist is licensed by the state.

◆ A marriage and family counselor has a Master's degree and is licensed by the state to perform marital counseling, although she may be trained in other disciplines.

A person with a Master's degree in social work is usually trained in psychotherapy and is licensed by the state as an licensed clinical social worker (L.C.S.W.).

Red Flag _____

> The vast majority of mental health professionals are ethical, competent, and extremely compassionate. However, as in any other profession, you will encounter the occasional "bad apple." If you or a loved one feel that a therapist has been unprofessional or incompetent or has otherwise neglected her duties, you can find another therapist. In cases of a breach of confidentiality or inappropriate sexual advances, you can report her to the appropriate state license board.

Pharmacological Therapy

This is the primary therapy you will need for bipolar disorder. You can get medication from a psychiatrist family doctor, or nurse practitioner, if trained in psychotropic drugs. More family doctors and nurse practitioners are getting involved in the treatment of bipolar disorder, as psychiatrists are becoming overburdened. In most areas of the country, there is no such thing as getting a quick appointment with a psychiatrist. Some family doctors are being trained to become the first doctor that someone with BP can see. A family doctor can usually see a person by the next day, even the same day in an emergency.

In serious cases, a family doctor may be able to prescribe drugs that will stabilize a person rather quickly and enable him to wait for an appointment with a psychiatrist. In milder cases, it may be an advantage for a family doctor, who is more familiar with the patient and the family than a psychiatrist, to be involved in treatment. An increasing trend is for the family doctor to work with the therapist to stabilize BP.

Interpersonal and Social Rhythm Therapy

Interpersonal and social rhythm therapy is an evidence-based hybrid therapy recommended by the National Institute of Mental Health (NIMH) and specially designed for bipolar disorder. The therapy approaches the bipolar problem from three different vantage points.

First, the client monitors her sleep. She keeps a sleep log and reports to the therapist. Sleep can be the most problematic area for someone with BP, so it stands to reason that this is an important aspect of therapy.

Second, consistent routines are an important aspect of treating BP. Having a routine, a purpose, and direction is a stabilizing factor for bipolar patients. The therapist works with the client to develop a daily routine, talk about a purpose in life, and provide direction.

Third, BP clients will find it a great benefit to learn interpersonal skills—tools for repairing relationships. Most people who have BP put dents in their relationships—big dents and little dents. They don't mean to. Tools for repairing relationships are a brilliant aspect of this therapy.

Cognitive Behavioral Therapy

Cognitive behavioral therapy was the first evidence-based therapy recommended by the NIMH. If it is specifically targeted toward bipolar disorder, it can help stabilize a person by helping him learn to change negative thought patterns and behaviors usually associated with BP.

The therapist might ask about a certain behavior, for example, and then ask about your beliefs behind that behavior.

You might write down the things that precipitated your last episode, so that if your lobe starts going out, you have something written to fall back on for guidance.

Psychoeducation

In psychoeducation, the therapist concentrates on the bipolar disorder, teaching about the disorder and the treatment, signs of reoccurrence, and so on. The client learns to recognize the signs.

The therapist may ask, "What precipitated your last episode?"

You might say, "I started buying cars and flirting."

Therapist: "Hmmm. Didn't you just buy a car?"

You: "Yes, as a matter of fact, I did."

Therapist: "Were you flirting with my secretary last week?"

You: "I guess I was!"

A discussion of why you bought the car or if you have been taking your medication or if something is happening in your life might follow.

Group Therapy

In addition to (and sometimes as a substitute for) one-on-one therapy, you may have the opportunity to participate in group therapy sessions. Group therapy has its good points and bad points. On the plus side, it's often helpful to discover that other people are facing the same problems and challenges as you are. You might learn a few effective techniques from hearing how they successfully handled certain situations. Some people also find therapy to be more comfortable when they're not always the one in the hot seat. In a group situation, you don't always feel like you're the one under the microscope.

On the other hand, group therapy can have its drawbacks, too. If you are going through a rough patch and have serious symptoms, the therapist may not be able to provide you with as much attention as you need. Plus, you may find it troubling or emotionally draining to hear about everyone else's problems—which can be especially problematic if you yourself aren't in the best state of mind at the moment.

One of the problems that therapists have with bipolar groups is that they spend a lot of time getting the group started only to have it dissipate a few months later. People come intermittently or quit. There is a secret to keeping the group going. The significant others and family should be invited and allowed to come even when the client doesn't come. There should be a therapy week and an education week. Groups set up like this may last for years. People with BP have a hard time staying at home with racing thoughts while their parents are at group talking about them.

Natural Therapy

These days, natural and holistic therapies are more popular than ever. Lots of people swear by natural remedies for all sorts of physical and psychological problems, but some in the traditional medical community are skeptical about the effectiveness of natural treatments.

This author is pro-natural. If there is a natural way to do something, I prefer to do that. One must remember, though, that "natural" does not necessarily mean "safe." Kava kava can affect your liver when used in high dosages, for example. (Heroin is natural, too, but I don't think that's good for you either!) I have searched high and low for naturopathic remedies for bipolar disorder and have not found any as reliable as prescription drugs. Still, it may be worth trying some of the safer natural treatments to see if you notice any benefits.

The most widely accepted natural treatment, researched and recommended by the

NIMH, is a daily dose of omega-3. The benefits of omega-3s are accepted by the medical community as well as the naturalists, and omega-3s have health benefits beyond the prevention of bipolar episodes. One psychiatrist recommends 7,500 to 11,000 mg per day during unstable periods and a maintenance dosage of 2,000 mg per day. Prescription-strength omega-3 is available as well and must be prescribed by a doctor. You should clear with your doctor any natural substance you want to take. Some of the natural things are contraindicated with some prescription medication.

The most natural medication for bipolar disorder that works is probably lithium. Valproic acid follows a close second.

Red Flag

While omega-3s can help reduce and prevent bipolar symptoms, they are not a substitute for prescription medications. The NIMH research shows that omega-3s prevent BP episodes by about 25 percent. Most doctors will tell you that they can be used along with medication, but check with your doctor: it may depend on the medication.

Electroconvulsive Therapy (ECT)

Electroconvulsive therapy (ECT) has been looked upon as barbaric by the public since it was first used in the 1930s. ECT's bad reputation is largely due to its portrayal in popular films, perhaps most famously in *One Flew Over the Cuckoo's Nest*. ECT is still used for severe depression. Many patients and doctors alike don't even want to consider this type of therapy.

But ECT is still used in some cases—especially in situations where the patient has reached a critical point and immediate, drastic action is necessary. Improvements have made it quite comfortable for the patient. Dr. Kay Jamison, named one of the "Best Doctors in the United States" and chosen by *Time* magazine as a "Hero of Medicine," says that ECT is sometimes the only thing that gets her out of her bipolar depression. Dr. Jamison is a tenured professor at Johns Hopkins University. Her most popular book for laypeople is called *An Unquiet Mind*.

Some doctors believe that ECT is safer than lithium. ECT can provide relatively immediate stabilization of severe mental illnesses. ECT is especially useful in cases when the patient is too ill to wait for medications to be effective. Patients with heart problems, pregnant patients who cannot take medications, and those who cannot tolerate drug treatments can be successfully and safely treated with ECT.

Today, the ECT procedure begins with the doctor giving you a muscle relaxant and a short-acting anesthetic. After you are relaxed, a small amount of electric current is sent to the left side of your head by way of electrodes. If this turns out to be ineffective, pads may be attached to both sides of your head. Either way, the electricity stimulates a brain seizure that lasts for about 40 seconds. You are then whisked away to a recovery room, where you may experience some side effects. For most people, these include confusion and short-term memory loss. You may also experience headache, nausea, muscle soreness, and heart arrhythmias. Most people report these effects to be mild to moderate and permanent memory loss is not likely, according to researchers.

Researchers are still trying to understand exactly why ECT helps people with mood disorders. One theory is that ECT may increase the permeability of the blood-brain barrier. The blood-brain barrier is the place where blood from the body is able to share nutrients with and take waste away from the cerebral spinal fluid (CSF) that circulates in and around the brain and spinal cord. The reason it is called a "barrier" is that only certain very small molecules are able to cross from the blood into the CSF and vice versa, which prevents contamination of the brain by foreign invaders. By increasing the number of molecules that have access to the brain, ECT may allow more medication to cross over into parts of the brain responsible for improved mood.

Another theory is that thyroid-related hormone changes occur as a result of ECT and the hormones travel to parts of the brain responsible for mood. Other studies suggest that dopamine levels rise in the brain and elevate mood. Regardless of which of these theories hold water, the therapeutic results of ECT are nearly immediate.

Whatever the reason, ECT done in conjunction with drug treatments can make the drug work better, so it often allows a patient to take less medication for months after the procedure. Research indicates that about 80 percent of ECT-treated patients are happy with the results.

Real People

One older woman said she experienced a depression that lasted for years. She said she had tried everything. None of the antidepressants seemed to help. Diet and exercise didn't help. Divorce didn't help (well, "maybe a little," she said with a smile). But nothing seemed to work until she got so desperate that she agreed to ECT. After a treatment, she would lose her short-term memory and feel confused for about 7 or 8 hours, but she felt better. After a few treatments, she said she didn't feel depressed. It has been five years and her depression has not returned. She said, "For me, it was the only thing that worked!"

Other Types of Therapy

Numerous other types of therapy have been used to treat BP. Not all of these are "official" treatments recommended by the medical community. Bipolar patients claim to have been helped by everything from magnetic therapy to medical marijuana. It's possible that these patients did indeed get some legitimate benefits from the therapies they tried, but it's also possible that they were simply experiencing a placebo effect.

In this author's experience, people with BP did seem to have benefited from marijuana, finding that it acts as a mood stabilizer. While at the Caron Foundation (one of the top three drug and alcohol rehabilitation facilities in the country), I noticed that most people who had smoked marijuana for a year or more had become lethargic and unambitious. I would see school records where a basketball player who had been active in extracurricular activities would become a couch potato after a year of using marijuana. But I didn't see that in people with BP and wondered if we should legalize marijuana to treat bipolar disorder.

Evidently, others thought the same thing, so the use of marijuana to treat BP was researched, and the study's findings were presented in 2007 at the International Conference on Bipolar Disorder in Pittsburgh, Pennsylvania. The results showed that people with bipolar disorder who smoke marijuana had more episodes than those who did not. I hate to dash any hopes, but I don't think it will be legalized for bipolar disorder anytime soon. Apparently there are better mood stabilizers and, unlike marijuana, your insurance will pay for them.

We don't claim to have all the answers. If an unconventional treatment relieves your bipolar symptoms and lets you enjoy a happier life, that's wonderful. Trying an unconventional treatment is a personal decision, one you must make for yourself with help from your loved ones and medical professionals. Keep in mind, there have always been surges of hopeful treatments in any disease or disorder. With bipolar disorder, new drugs have been hyped up by drug companies, miracle natural remedies or therapies reported. They tend to peter out. No matter how well-meaning the purporters were, there always seems to be a catch. It could be a side effect or a long-term show stopper. That's why my recommendation is to rely on the drugs and therapies that we know about and have proven themselves (even with some uncomfortable side effects) until these new "miracle" discoveries prove themselves.

Finding a Therapist

So you've decided to give therapy a try. How do you find a therapist? Here are a few options:

◆ Contact your local Mental Health Association. Find out when the bipolar group meets. Go, then ask people in the group for therapist recommendations.

◆ Ask around. Check with friends and relatives to see if they can recommend anyone. These days, people see therapists for all sorts of things, and the concept of therapy is more socially accepted than in the past, so people may be more willing to discuss their experiences.

◆ Consult your doctor. You can ask your regular doctor for a referral to a good therapist in your area.

◆ Surf the web. The American Psychiatric Association's "Choosing a Psychiatrist" (available online as a PDF file) is an excellent source of advice. There are also online bipolar support groups and discussion boards where you can ask for recommendations.

◆ Check the Yellow Pages. The psychologists, counselors, or mental health groups listed may mention their treatment specialties.

◆ One way to get the best doctors is to call the nearest renowned teaching hospital and ask for a recommendation. If your bipolar disorder is complicated, call the best hospitals in the country and get ready to travel (Johns Hopkins, USC, Stanford, University of Pittsburgh Medical, University of Pennsylvania, and so on).

What to Expect

It's natural to be anxious before your first therapy session, especially if you don't know what to expect. Therapy is a highly individualized situation, so everyone's experience will be a little different. But here are some things to expect:

◆ Plan on spending a sizable portion of the first session (and perhaps more after that) telling your therapist your background. This includes your medical history, all of your BP-related experiences, past traumas, and other important experiences in your life.

- You may not be understood completely, at least at first. Expect that you *will* be understood enough to be helped.

- Don't expect instant results. Therapy can be a slow process. You should, however, see steady and gradual improvements as therapy progresses.

Mental Note

The patient/therapist relationship is a partnership, and it's important that both partners feel comfortable with each other. If you find that you don't click with your therapist (for whatever reason), don't be afraid to switch to another therapist who is a better match.

Support Groups

Support groups can also be an important part of a bipolar treatment plan. Many people with BP consider their support group or groups to be a lifesaver.

The Depression and Bipolar Support Alliance (DBSA) and the National Alliance on Mental Illness (NAMI) are the two main national support groups. Check their websites for information about local resources and meetings in your area. There are also plenty of smaller local support groups. Ask your therapist for recommendations, or check your phone book for mental health organizations and resources in your area.

If you can't find any groups in your area—or if you prefer to remain somewhat anonymous—there are also bipolar support groups online, which you can find easily by using a search engine.

Family Therapy

It seems that the most successful therapy includes the patient's family and significant other. Certainly there will be times when the patient should see the therapist or doctor alone and confidentially. But family involvement, directed by the therapist or doctor, seems to be very helpful in many cases. Feedback from family members can be very valuable and can even be the difference between life and death. In addition, the therapist can help your loved ones understand what you are going through, and together all of you can figure out ways that you and your friends and family can have happy, positive relationships.

Family therapy is an evidence-based therapy and is recommended by the NIMH for bipolar disorder.

The Least You Need to Know

♦ Therapy is a critical part of a BP treatment plan.

♦ For best results, your treatment plan should include a combination of medication and therapy.

♦ There are several different types of therapy for BP. It's okay to try a few until you find the treatment that best augments your medical therapy and that works best for you.

♦ When you are able to talk to someone confidentially with no fear of being judged and no fear of it being repeated, it can be a tremendous relief.

13

Lifestyle Changes

In This Chapter

- ◆ Enlightening insights into bipolar disorder
- ◆ A method of change
- ◆ Cruising on autopilot with a routine

If you've recently been diagnosed with bipolar disorder—or are struggling to get your bipolar disorder under control—it's important to examine your lifestyle and habits. Some lifestyle changes may be necessary to keep your moods and symptoms under control. In this chapter, we'll address some of those lifestyle issues and suggest changes you can make.

Difficult but Important Lifestyle Changes

Anyone who has ever tried to lose 5 pounds knows how difficult it is to make a consistent change to one's eating and exercise habits, even for a week or two. Now imagine trying to lose 200 pounds without the help of a personal trainer, a dietician, a gastric surgeon, or appetite-suppressing drugs. Who can do that?

Probably no one. Like an obese person who cannot stop eating, a bipolar person often cannot control the powerful impulses and compulsions that drive his unhealthy behaviors. Without help, the major lifestyle changes needed to properly manage the symptoms of the disorder may be relatively impossible to achieve.

Lifestyle is important because the way you live has a lot of influence over how you feel. Most people with BP become accustomed to just "getting by," rather than really living life before they are diagnosed and treated. Control over the disorder is essential to maintain control of your life and allows you the freedom to make healthy decisions.

Health Through Lifestyle

Most of our habits are things we enjoy, although we may have some habits we don't really like doing but find difficult to stop. To structure a healthy lifestyle, you may have to make a lot of changes to your habits. Typical onset for bipolar symptoms is between the ages of 15 and 25. Smoking, drinking, using drugs to self-medicate, and behaving recklessly may be well-established habits in the lives of bipolar people by the time they are diagnosed. Changing these habits can take tremendous effort, but relearning how to live can help bipolar sufferers avoid many major problems.

We discussed some ways you can establish a healthy lifestyle in Chapter 10, where we presented the six "-ates." In this chapter, we will introduce you to the three "-aces": face, replace, and pace.

Face

Take a good long look in the mirror. Be honest with yourself. Identify what you like and what you don't like. Consider your abilities and your shortcomings. Make a list of your positives and your negatives. Envision who you would like to be, where you would like to be, what you would like to be.

It doesn't matter how old you are or where you live. Self-improvement is achievable. First, though, you must arrive at your short-term and long-term goals. Perhaps you would like to go back to school and make a career change. Perhaps you want to start sailing or learn to fly a plane. Maybe you want to move somewhere sunnier or re-establish and re-energize your relationships with your spouse, children, or parents. Realize what things are important to you and try to rank them in order from most important to least. Then consider what actions you will have to take to achieve those goals.

Let's say you want to become a marathon runner. The first thing you realize is that you'll have to stop smoking. The long-term goal is to become a runner; the short-term goal is to stop smoking and improve your lung function. Think of a plan to quit smoking. Your plan should include getting a physical and getting the okay from your doctor to begin taking short runs. Maybe she will suggest you try the nicotine patch to curb your smoking while you start getting in shape.

Sometimes, the very act of establishing a bigger goal makes obstacles seem smaller. If you don't have a place you want to get to, you will probably end up somewhere else.

Replace

It is much easier to stop one habit if you put another in its place. Many of the problems of the bipolar lifestyle are centered on the use of drugs and alcohol. Once you begin your medication regimen under the supervision of your doctor, your reliance on self-medication should be much easier to end.

Think about how drugs and alcohol fit into your routine. Think about how they have affected your life and decide if they should still have a place in it. If your first stop after work was the local watering hole, where you liked to be around a group of your friends, it may not be easy for you to stop there and drink soda. It won't be the same as it was when you were drinking alcohol along with them. You can choose instead to go to the gym and unwind with some physical activity like swimming or aerobics and meet some new friends. You can't replace your old friends, but you can meet new ones with whom you can engage in healthy activities.

You can choose to feel better over feeling worse. Think about how you feel when you get up with a headache and an empty wallet in the morning and drag yourself to work. Think about how good you might feel in the morning after swimming laps the night before and eating a healthy dinner. You can choose to replace smoking while you watch TV at night with knitting. You can learn to play a musical instrument instead of watching TV.

Think about the things you have always wanted to do, if only you had more time. If you decide to pursue one of these interests instead of some bad habit, you might be able to create a new habit. Replace activities, don't just resolve to quit them. Idle hands are the devil's workshop, and the best way to commit to a new routine is to plan one.

Pace

Pace yourself in your pursuit of a new lifestyle. It doesn't have to happen overnight. You can go to the bar after work one night and say hello to your friends. The next day after work, you can go to the gym or do some volunteer work, like walking the dogs at the local shelter, before going home. If you start taking guitar lessons a few nights a week, it will surely cut down on your time smoking in front of the TV.

Take your time learning a new skill or pursuing your interests. Make sure the activity you choose is something that you will enjoy doing even if you aren't good at it. You will still find relaxation and satisfaction in it if you do it at a realistic pace.

Sleep

A *circadian rhythm* is a roughly 24-hour cycle in the biochemical, physiological, and behavioral processes of human beings. A number of disorders, including bipolar disorder, are associated with irregular or pathological functioning of circadian rhythms. Recent research suggests that circadian rhythm disturbances found in bipolar disorder are positively influenced by lithium's effect on clock genes (your internal clock mechanism, the genetic component of the mammalian clock, a protein known as "Rora").

A book on social rhythm therapy will usually include a sleep log that is appropriate for people with BP. Social rhythm is a hybrid therapy designed specifically for people with BP.

def•i•ni•tion

The term *circadian*, coined by Franz Halberg, comes from the Latin *circa*, "around," and *diem*, "day," and literally means "approximately one day."
Circadian rhythms allow organisms to anticipate and prepare for precise and regular environmental changes.

 Red Flag

Seasonal affective disorder (SAD) is driven by light. About 20 percent of people who experience depression due to SAD may go on to develop symptoms of bipolar disorder. It's important to discern between recovery from winter depression and a manic episode because the treatment is different. People with BP and SAD may experience depression during the winter and hypomania in the summer.

Daily Routine

A daily routine is tantamount to a happy bipolar life. People who are bipolar think out of the box, but they need a box to think out of. In Chapter 23, we talk about bipolar kids and how important it is to have a routine. (You can peek ahead if you want. Aw, go ahead. I know you want to. Meet us back here.)

Imagine that your prefrontal lobe goes out and you don't have a routine. How do you know what to do next? How do you plan your day? People with BP usually don't like it when their plans go awry. Not having a plan could be even worse, and not being able to make a plan worse yet. When your lobe goes out, you may feel a little out of touch with reality, but at least you know you go to the gym every day at 6 P.M. That gives you a sense of stability. Maybe you shouldn't have had that 100 percent Kona coffee earlier. You probably felt like the big kahuna for a while, but look at you now. You almost made a wrong turn coming to the gym.

This is why a routine is important. It helps orient you after the surprise Kona hangover temporarily shuts down some neurons in your prefrontal lobe. Exercise at the gym, go home, and make sure you get enough sleep tonight. I hear they have some decaffeinated Kona that tastes the same. Try that tomorrow with your breakfast Pop Tart (but first, see "Sugar" in the "Diet" section of this chapter).

Stress

As you no doubt already know, stress can cause all sorts of physical and emotional problems. Stress can be caused by external factors (noise, a chaotic work environment, traffic) or by internal factors like worry and anxiety (whether the cause of the anxiety is real or imagined).

Stress is especially risky for people with mood disorders, for many reasons. It can upset your already-delicate chemical state, disrupt your sleep cycle, affect how your medications work, and cause lots of other complications.

Here's the tricky part: how do you avoid stress? Well, unfortunately it's nearly impossible to totally avoid it, but you can try to avoid situations that are guaranteed to be very stressful—for example, confrontations with people you don't get along with.

Since you can't avoid stress completely, it's important that you learn to handle it with therapy, exercise, meditation, and so on. This can help calm your system and minimize the physical and emotional fallout.

Diet

A healthy diet low in saturated fats and rich in whole grains, fresh fruits, and vegetables is important. People with bipolar disorder should maintain a regular healthy diet, restricting calories if they are on medications that cause weight gain.

Research indicates that omega-3 fatty acids found in fish such as mackerel, sardines, salmon, and bluefish may help reduce and prevent symptoms of bipolar disorder. Researchers from NIMH have investigated the effects of supplements of the omega-3 fatty acids EPA and DHA for patients who have BP. People who have a good omega-3 diet have reduced episodes by 25 percent.

Sugar

Many people use sugar—especially sweets like chocolate—as a comfort or coping mechanism. Here's something you may not know: high sugar intake can actually contribute to depression. Sure, that "sugar high" might make you feel good for a short time, but it's often followed by a crash, which can send your mood plunging. Keeping your sugar intake steady at a reasonable level will also keep your insulin levels regulated, which helps keep your moods stable.

Caffeine

Any psychostimulant is contraindicated (a no-no) with bipolar disorder. That includes anything with caffeine in it (coffee, tea, chocolate, caffeinated soda). Decaffeinated coffee can be brewed and tastes the same, without the buzz.

Keep in mind that every time you take in a psychostimulant, or drink alcohol, or do a recreational drug, it's like prodding the bipolar monster with a stick. Pray that you don't wake up the bipolar monster. The monster is either going to sit on you (depression), or go on a rampage trying to wreck your life (mania experienced as euphoria, rage, irritability, or agitation).

Exercise

A study of 21 individual bipolar cases showed that exercise reduced and possibly prevented bipolar symptoms. In one case, a young woman said she had to be careful of the "runner's high," as the endorphins started to trigger some mania. She makes sure she slows down when she feels it coming on.

One young man, calling himself "bipolar extraordinaire," said that his mother encouraged a lot of physical activity for him in high school. He ran every morning and went out for several different sports. He believes that the exercise delayed his first full-blown manic episode, which he had in college when he was getting very little physical activity.

One important factor in exercise is to put limits on it. Exercising "in the morning" could mean *all* morning on a manic day and could lead to injury. Set a routine for exercise between certain times, and set a time limit.

Alcohol and Marijuana

Many people with BP use alcohol to reduce racing thoughts and agitation and to calm down. It may also be used as a sleep aid. A certain amount of alcohol can make a person with BP hypomanic. What a wonderful medication, yes? No. In the long run, it causes depression, addiction, and even bad breath.

What about marijuana? It acts as a mood stabilizer. It slows down racing thoughts. It calms a person down and reduces agitation. Should it be legalized for people with BP? As stated in another chapter, researchers were starting to think that way, but it turns out that people who use marijuana have an increased number of episodes in the long run. Some people will be very disappointed to find this out. Don't write a nasty letter to the messenger.

The physical environment probably doesn't matter as much as the psychological environment for people with BP. It is important to have your team of consultants to call on when you need them. Your doctor, therapist, educated spouse, and trusted friends all comprise a healthy psychological environment.

The Least You Need to Know

- Lifestyle changes can be difficult but very beneficial.
- When you address the lifestyle issues necessary for controlling bipolar disorder, your life can change for the better.
- What you ingest and what you do can have a significant effect on how you feel and how you function.
- Drugs and alcohol are not good medications, even if Grandma imbibed some (for medicinal purposes only, of course).

Chapter 14

Hospitalization

In This Chapter

- ◆ Why you may need hospitalization
- ◆ Involuntary versus voluntary commitment
- ◆ What will happen during your hospital stay

In a perfect scenario, a treatment plan including medication and therapy would keep your bipolar disorder under control. But sometimes things get more serious and you need to be hospitalized. In this chapter, we'll discuss what to do when you reach that point and how to make your hospital stay go as well as possible.

When Hospitalization Is Necessary

Hospitalization is necessary when you are a danger to yourself or others. Chronic suicidal or homicidal thoughts, or thoughts of hurting yourself or others, warrant a visit to the hospital. In fact, under these conditions, the law says you have to go. Experts in crisis intervention will determine whether you need to become an inpatient at the hospital or if you can be treated as an outpatient.

Most hospitals prefer to treat patients on an outpatient basis, except in cases when the patient or those in contact with the patient are clearly in danger. It is also sometimes necessary to become an inpatient if you can't take care of yourself or your dependents, such as your children or elderly parents. Again, the intake experts at the mental health facility will make this determination.

The important thing is to recognize when a hospital evaluation is a good idea. When you are very mentally ill, you may not be fully aware of the severity of your situation. You may not be able to properly weigh the risk you pose to yourself or others. As a general rule, you are considered dangerous to yourself or others if any of the following criteria apply:

◆ You have made threats to another or attempted to inflict harm or have inflicted harm on someone. It may be a better option for you to go to the hospital rather than jail if you are showing severe symptoms of bipolar disorder.

◆ You are unable to meet your own basic needs (or those of dependent minors) for food, personal hygiene, health care, housing, and personal safety and there is a "reasonable probability" of serious physical harm coming to you without care and supervision.

◆ You have attempted or threatened to commit suicide and there is "reasonable probability" that you will make a suicide attempt without care and supervision.

◆ You have mutilated or attempted to mutilate yourself (or others) and there is a "reasonable probability" another attempt will be made without care and supervision.

◆ You are incapable of exercising self-control or of making sound judgments in conducting the responsibilities of everyday life without care and supervision in such a way that you are a danger to yourself or others.

Types of Hospital Commitments

Let's learn some important terms associated with inpatient treatment: involuntary commitment and voluntary commitment.

Involuntary Commitment

Patients with Bipolar I disorder who have experienced a full-blown manic episode are often hospitalized at some point. Since acute manic episodes disturb insight and judgment, individuals with mania are often hospitalized against their will, which is referred to as *involuntary commitment*. Involuntary commitments can be very extremely unsettling for patients and their loved ones. However, most people are later grateful that they were forced into treatment.

In most states, an involuntary commitment requires that a person be harmful to himself or to others. This could involve suicidal or homicidal threats. It could involve unsanitary living conditions or lack of care for oneself.

For example, an incarcerated woman refused medication. She had a physical problem for which she also refused treatment. The situation became so dangerous that a hearing was held at the jail and the doctor, nurse, psychologist, and psychiatrist testified. The public attorney representing her did not have much of a case for her refusal. The judge ordered treatment and the woman was strapped down and given medication for her mental disorder, until she was compliant enough for her physical problem to be treated. It took four corrections officers to contain her.

Three days later, when the woman was in her right mind, she said to the psychologist, "I guess I really gave you guys a run for your money. I'm sorry, and thank you for helping me. I just get like that without my medication." She had been taking her medication regularly for years, but due to a mix-up, her psychiatrist had gone on vacation for a month without ordering a mandatory white blood cell count. The drug store could not dispense her medication.

After a week without medication, she wandered off from her home in West Virginia and ended up incarcerated in Pennsylvania for criminal trespassing. Once she was able to communicate, her family was notified. She had been missing for months and had three children who were waiting for her. When she was on her medication, she was perfectly able to function. The charges were dropped and she went back home to her family.

def•i•ni•tion

Involuntary commitment is when you are admitted to a hospital or psychiatric treatment facility against your will.

The procedures for involuntary commitments vary by state. We advise that you look online or go to your local law library to find information specific to your state for your own protection and edification.

Involuntary commitment must be ordered by a judge in the case of a long-term incarceration at a mental facility. It requires at least one mental-health professional and the state court to agree that you need to be there. For short-term incarcerations, a doctor or law enforcement officer can order that you be held and evaluated, against your will if necessary, for a 24-hour period. If, during those 24 hours, you are found to be a danger to yourself or others, they may ask the court to commit you for an additional few days to stabilize you.

Mental Note _____

The National Association of Psychiatric Health Systems reports that about 22 percent of adults treated in its members' hospitals are admitted involuntarily.

Involuntary commitments are intended to help you receive necessary and appropriate mental health or substance abuse treatment. Abuses of these otherwise lifesaving laws probably occurred more often in the past than they do today. Today, doctors must testify to the court about your condition, and you are joined by counsel in your defense and family members who support you. If you cannot afford an attorney for such a proceeding, one will be appointed for you. In court, an impartial judge listens to both sides and determines if an involuntary stay at a facility is required.

These days there are many protections for the mentally ill that did not exist just a few decades ago. However, in most mishandled commitment cases (past or present), the victims of unwarranted involuntary incarcerations had no family or friends involved on their behalf. This is why you should appoint loved ones to advocate for you, whether you are recovering from a cardiac triple bypass or a severe mental illness. The Mental Patient's Bill of Rights is usually available from the state offices of the attorney general and usually online. You may wish to avail yourself and your advocates of these rights.

Voluntary Commitment

If you are very ill and prefer to focus solely on becoming well, a hospital stay may be the right thing for you. Imagine: no cooking, no cleaning, no work deadlines, no traffic jams, no interference by well-meaning worrywarts or nosy Nellies. Nothing but you and an entire team of pros working to alleviate your mental suffering. Sounds kind of like a vacation from regular life, doesn't it? Well, it is, and it can be the fastest route to a healthy, productive life on your own.

Unlike in an involuntary commitment, you decide that you want to reside for a time at a facility of your choice, and you are free to leave the facility even against the advice of medical personnel. In most places you do have to provide a period of notice for administrative purposes and discharge instructions. Sometimes the facility may require that you leave during daylight hours. Rules like these are mainly measures to reduce liability to the hospital by your leaving.

If you leave AMA (against medical advice), your insurance may not pay and you may be required to pay the hospital bill. It is best to just let them take care of you. If you are a danger to yourself or others, the hospital may formally begin involuntary procedures. Like we said, it is best to just let them take care of you.

In Chapter 19 we will detail a legal document known as an *advance directive*, in which you can, in advance, consent to special conditions of voluntary admission to a hospital and thus avoid involuntary commitment.

Mental Note _____

The period of notice required before you leave a treatment facility gives the hospital time to begin involuntary commitment procedures against you if you meet the criteria for involuntary commitment.

Choosing the Right Hospital—and Affording It

If you decide that hospitalization is the best choice for you, you have many treatment options. These choices may include …

- Inpatient care in general hospital psychiatric units.

- Private psychiatric hospitals.

- State and federal public psychiatric hospitals.

- Veterans Administration (VA) hospitals.

- Community mental health centers.

- Partial hospitalization programs.

Things you should consider when deciding which facility is right for you include geography, cost, type of treatment, and who might attend to your business while you are away. New York, California, and Florida boast some of the most reputable, cutting-edge, mental health treatment centers in the nation if you can travel. If you need to be on hand geographically, your options may be limited.

The Price/Insurance Issue

Blessed with great insurance benefits or enough bucks of your own? Then the sky is the limit. You may opt to get well among the rich and famous at a hospital that resembles a resort. If you have health insurance, contact your insurance company and find out about your coverage and its limitations. You may have to choose from facilities within your insurer's network if you don't want to pay for the care yourself.

If you are uninsured or underinsured, you can choose among nonprofit, community, state, and federal hospitals that offer free services or fees based on your income (sliding-scale services). You may have to wait for a bed to open up in some states with limited resources. There are many providers of quality care in every state, so if you have the means you can decide if you are willing to travel to the facility that is best for you or if distance is a limiting factor.

You should also consider how long you might be able to stay in the hospital. Currently, the average stay for an adult patient in a psychiatric facility is 12 days. With that in mind, think about dependable persons you might rely on to mind your affairs while you are away. If you are responsible for a dependent and have no one able to care for him or her, contact your local social services office and ask about respite agencies in the area.

By the time you need help, you may be unable to make these choices and decisions. Let us stress, once more, that you should think this through with a trusted friend, therapist, spouse, or medical doctor *before* you have an episode.

Typical Costs

To give you an idea of the costs associated with hospitalization, fees for inpatients in 24-hour care commonly range from $400 to $550 per day. Partial hospitalizations, such as day-treatment programs, are quite similar to inpatient hospital care and range from $95 to $175 per day. (These rates are approximate for 2008.) The rates may depend on which part of the country you are in and the rising cost of care. Community health centers are typically the least expensive options, often offer residential and day programs, and are usually free to residents of the community.

Researching Facilities

See Appendix B for a comprehensive list of directories of accredited facilities by state. If you plan to search for local public or private services, check the Yellow Pages for your branch of the Mental Health Association (MHA) or call the National Mental Health Association at (800) 969-NMHA for the address of your local branch. The MHA can also provide contact information for all the hospitals near you.

What to Expect

In both hospitals and care centers, you will receive treatment based on a plan developed by your assigned psychiatrist. The therapies outlined in that plan will likely involve a variety of other mental health professionals, such as a clinical psychologist, nursing staff, social workers, rehabilitation therapists, and addiction counselors.

Inpatient treatment usually cannot begin until a physical examination is performed. After that, formal treatment begins, usually one-on-one with a primary therapist every day. Group therapy will also be a daily event. In therapy sessions, you will learn about your illness, yourself, your life, and the people in your life. You will be taught tools for managing your feelings, your life, and your relationships. Often you will begin a regimen of psychiatric medications right away. The hospital personnel will pay careful attention to your physical well-being. Physicians and nurses will monitor you for adverse reactions to medications as well as for therapeutic effects.

The hospital offers a safe environment where you can focus on becoming well without the stresses of everyday life. In most cases, due to improved psychotherapy and new medications, it doesn't take very long to stabilize a mental illness and get back on the road to recovery.

Once your condition is relatively stable, you may choose to move to a less-intensive treatment setting, such as partial hospitalization or a community health center. Both offer programs that provide psychotherapy, assistance with educational or occupational needs, and other services that will help you function at home, at work, and in social circles. In these programs, your friends and family can help monitor your progress because you can return home at night and on weekends.

Here's a hospitalization checklist for both people who are already receiving treatment, as well as for newbies.

Things to take:

◆ Your favorite comfortable clothes and pajamas and shoes or slippers without laces, so you don't have to wear hospital garb. (Laces aren't usually allowed in hospital settings as a standard suicide prevention. Even if you are not at risk of suicide, someone else may be.)

◆ Your own pillow and blankets. They will most likely be more comfortable than those the facility offers.

◆ All medications you take, including dietary supplements and over-the-counter products you use regularly. The staff will need to see what you are taking and the amounts. (In a rehab facility, you may be issued new medications and not allowed to take in your own, because illegal drugs can be smuggled in that way.)

◆ The phone numbers of the psychiatrist, therapist, and any other mental health professionals you are seeing. The hospital may want your records from them or to ask them questions.

- Reading material, playing cards, and pictures of people and pets (without frames) to make it cozier.

- A note pad (without wires or spirals) in which you can keep a journal. Before you go, write the phone numbers of your doctors and friends and family members in it, in case your treatments or medication give you memory problems.

- Cigarettes if you smoke and chewing gum if you don't. Almost everyone in a psych ward smokes, so it isn't the best place or time to attempt to quit.

- Take this book with you.

Things not to take:

- Anything valuable, because it could get lost, stolen, or forgotten. Leave jewelry and large sums of cash at home or in the bank (or send them to the author of this book).

- Anything sharp or that can cut or poke, such as pencils, knives, tweezers, or mirrors.

- Shoelaces, belts, or anything that could be used by someone with suicidal tendencies.

- A cell phone or computer. You probably won't be allowed to use them.

Mental Note

Don't let these rules scare you. They are just normal precautions for everyone's safety.

Before you go (or as early in your stay as possible), ask about your phone privileges and when visitors are permitted. Touch base frequently with someone who will keep track of how you are doing and keep you posted on what is going on at home.

Here are a few other things you should know about your hospital stay:

- In most hospitals you will share a room with another patient. Don't expect the same privacy you have at home!

- Your time in the hospital will be on a schedule. Breakfast, lunch, and dinner will be served at specific times. Group therapy and individual therapy sessions, as well as free time and bedtimes, are all scheduled.

◆ You are not required to participate in group activities, but you may miss out on some of the benefits of your stay if you don't. You may be required to attend, but you are not required to speak. In most hospitals you may invite your family to group sessions, thereby involving them in your treatment.

◆ In extreme situations, such as a psychotic episode, the caregivers may take steps to protect you from injury, including the use of restraints for brief periods.

The Least You Need to Know

◆ Hospitalization, while usually a last resort, can sometimes be the most effective way to get your BP under control quickly.

◆ If you are deemed a danger to yourself or others, you may be committed to a hospital or other treatment facility without your consent.

◆ Your hospital options will depend on your location, insurance coverage, and ability to pay.

◆ The first admission to the hospital appears more dreadful than it actually is, and if you ever need to be admitted again, you'll be much less reluctant.

Part 4

Living With Bipolar Disorder

As you probably already know, bipolar disorder affects all aspects of your life. In this part, we will talk about how you can live—happily and productively—with bipolar disorder. From employment to family life, we will share advice that we hope will make your life a little bit easier to manage.

15

What to Expect

In This Chapter

- ◆ General expectations about having BP
- ◆ Questions to ask yourself to ward off an episode
- ◆ What to expect with age
- ◆ The kindling effect with age

If you've recently been diagnosed with bipolar disorder (or are just now coming to terms with a previous diagnosis), you may be wondering exactly what you are in for. In this chapter, we'll try to give you a realistic idea of what you can expect your life with BP to be like. Everyone is different and everyone may be affected differently, but some general aspects of BP affect most people.

Living Your Life

Each person with BP has his or her own symptoms. They may be similar to those of others with BP, but will not be exactly the same for everyone. There are four chromosomal regions suspected to be involved in bipolar disorder, which means there may be at least 16 different types of bipolar disorder. How the disease affects a person also depends on how many chromosomal regions are "turned on" on any given day: hopefully none.

Getting Through the Days

Prodromal symptoms (early indications of an episodic onset) may include depressed mood, hopelessness, increased (or decreased) energy, irritability, anger or quickness to anger, conduct problems, bold behavior, and hypersensitivity to criticism or rejection.

Depression is one of the usual symptoms of BP. The bipolar monster falls asleep with its heavy head on your chest. If depression lasts the whole day instead of just part of the day, it may be time to do something about it. Some people have to push the bipolar monster off each day before they get out of bed. Once they've thrown the monster on their bedroom floor, they usually start to feel better.

Some people go through long periods, even years, of no symptoms. Other people have a low-level depression every day that may or may not be due to BP. Many people experience mania first. It may appear as euphoria, agitation, or anger.

Let's look at some scenarios of daily life. Bipolar disorder can magnify your feelings. You may be tapping your foot, for example, and someone may say, "Could you stop doing that?"

Your mind may blow the comment way out of proportion and you may think, "I must be annoying to him. That's what I am—one big annoyance! Who does he think he is, anyway? He has faults, too!"

So then you say, "Fine! I'll stop tapping my foot, if you stop criticizing me for everything I do!"

You don't have to be bipolar to have this happen, but if you notice that you are taking everything personally, it may be a sign that you are overreacting.

Inability to sleep is another big sign. Many people with BP have an ongoing problem with sleep. As we have said before, sleep problems may be the biggest indicator and cause of worsening bipolar symptoms. If you are having trouble sleeping, do something about it right away. Cancel your late night out. Ask your doctor about taking a little more medication temporarily. Do your sleep exercises. Go for a massage to relax. Other people may not understand why you have to cancel the party at the last minute, or why it's so important for you to go for a massage, but you need to do what you have to do to balance your life.

Getting the Understanding You Need

You may run into a lack of understanding from people who do not know much about bipolar disorder. Most people, in fact, do not understand BP, and that makes it all the more challenging. Let's say your boss asks you to work the midnight shift for a couple weeks to cover for someone on vacation. Can you do it? No, you can't. You can say you're sorry and you can't say why, but you can get your boss a doctor's note if she needs one.

When the majority of people do not understand bipolar disorder, it may be best to keep it private even with your boss. The best advice is to divulge the information on a "need to know" basis. If your boss ever needs to know because you end up in a psych ward for a week, tell him then or just before you go and remind him it is a confidential medical problem. If you have a good rapport with your boss and you don't think he will hold it against you, then tell him that you have bipolar disorder and the interruption in circadian rhythm can propel you into a manic episode if you work midnight shift. So if he doesn't want you to dye your hair green in a manic episode, he will ask someone else.

Real People

A woman was working in a child-care facility. The children loved her and she loved her job. During a stressful period, she called her doctor and said, "I think my medication needs to be adjusted. I am getting racing thoughts and I'm afraid I'll be so preoccupied with my thoughts that I won't be able to give the children my full attention. If I feel this way tomorrow, I won't be able to go to work. Should I tell my manager I have bipolar disorder?"

The doctor said, "No. Tell them something they will understand. Come into my office tomorrow and I will adjust your medication."

The woman called in sick the next day with "hormonal" problems. (Dopamine is a hormone, isn't it?) Her boss understood that.

There may be peaks and valleys during your day. Many people with BP recognize that mornings are not their best time of day. One BP boss told his employees that it might be better if they could wait until the afternoon if they needed to come and talk to him. Of course, some employees didn't take heed, and when they went to talk to him in the morning it was like going into a verbal slaughterhouse. His voice could be heard throughout the office, shouting, "What?! You want a vacation day tomorrow?! And you're telling me this *now?!*" But in the afternoon, he would go back to the employee and say, "Okay, I found someone to cover for you. Go ahead and take tomorrow off."

This same boss knew himself well and would not make any big decisions in the morning. If an executive called him in the morning, he would tell the executive he would get back to her in the afternoon.

Making It Work for You

Bipolar disorder is not fair. It doesn't care how it affects your daily life. It just is what it is. There are some things in life that you won't be able to do, but there are plenty of things you can do.

One man says he is grateful for having bipolar disorder. Before he realized he had the disorder, he was staying up until all hours of the morning, drinking and getting into trouble. Once he realized he had bipolar disorder, he knew he couldn't drink and he couldn't interfere with his sleep cycle. That made him unavailable to his rowdy friends. He started taking care of himself and made new friends. He started taking college courses at night, which was a better challenge than riding the electric bull at the bar. He feels the best he has ever felt and has a future now. His friends are supportive instead of bringing him down. He feels like his true self.

Important Things to Know

If you notice that your life is not working as well as it used to, it may be time to do a bipolar checklist. We have provided one with standard things to check for here, but you may want to add your own personal checks (or send the author a personal check).

One question to ask yourself is "What precipitated my last episode?" Maybe you started obsessing about making your appointments. Maybe you started spending too much money. Maybe your friends felt that you were being rude. You will have your own special signs besides the list of questions that follow:

◆ How much sleep have you gotten recently? Have you slept eight hours or more? Has your sleep been restless? Have you taken your sleep medication?*

◆ Have you been taking your medication? Do you have a way to know you have been taking it, such as a weekly pill box? Memory is not always reliable. Do you have someone checking your medication or giving it to you? Is your medication becoming less effective? Do you need to take more temporarily?*

◆ Do you find yourself getting impatient with people who talk too slowly? Do you finish other people's sentences?

◆ Are you impatient about waiting in line?

- Are you driving too fast? Do you cut people off?

- Do you feel overwhelmed by all the things you have to do? Are you unable to prioritize the important things first?

- Do you have too many goals? Are you thinking of even more goals?

- Do you have a really hard time getting out of bed in the morning?

- If you stop and think about it, is there something that is really stressing you out?

- Are your emotions magnified? Does your anger get triggered suddenly with your family or friends?

- Are you having too many sexual or romantic thoughts? Are you hypersexual?

- Are you worried about things you don't normally worry about?

- Are you checking everything (the calendar, things in the house, where people are, and so on) to excess?

- Are you getting a bit paranoid? Do you think your spouse is cheating on you? Do you think people are taking advantage of you without having any specific evidence?

- Are you doing things without taking the consequences into consideration?

- Do you feel agitated most of the day?

- Has something big happened to get you upset?

- Do you feel exhausted and at the same time energized?

- Are you hypervigilant (shaking your foot, tapping your fingers, or repeatedly swallowing, blinking, shrugging, and so on)?

- Has anything happened recently that may be a stressor? (These may include moving, separation, breaking off a relationship, a death, work problems, a job change, relationship problems, changing time zones, working another shift, legal problems, or money problems.)

- Do you feel like you are a robot, just going through the motions of life?

- Do you feel hopeless most of the time?

- Do people ask you to repeat yourself? Are you talking too fast or is your voice volume too low?

- Is your self-esteem too low or too high?

◆ Are you drinking too much or smoking marijuana or using other drugs?

◆ Have you had any appetite changes (not eating or overeating)?

◆ Are you fatigued?

◆ Are you doing anything that you did before your last episode? What precipitated your last episode?

These are some of the standard questions to ask yourself to anticipate an episode. It would be a good idea to involve a trusted friend or spouse in answering these questions or even ask him or her to sit down and ask you these questions. If you're on the verge of having some kind of major bipolar problem, your judgment may not be at its best, and someone who knows you may be able to help. The good news is that if you catch it early enough, you can usually avoid an episode.

As we have said before, you may have to call in your team (your doctor, your therapist, trusted people in your life) to avoid getting worse. The two biggest factors in precipitating an episode are getting enough sleep and taking your medication (see the asterisks on the preceding questions).

Real People

One woman knew enough to call her doctor and say, "I feel too good today!" In other words, she was manic. She was all too familiar with what happens next when she doesn't do anything about that addictive nice feeling. She had met a man she was attracted to and that stimulated her mania. Unfairly, this sometimes happens when a person with BP becomes sexually attracted. She knew herself, and she knew what the outcome of her good feelings would be, having played the situation out several times before.

What Round Is This?

As your bipolar disorder emerges, it reveals itself. You get to know it. Fights are won by professionals who study their opponents. Study your own bipolar disorder. Know thy enemy.

Ding! The bell goes off. If it's your first round with a bipolar episode, you might ask, "What was that ding sound?" You are easy prey for the bipolar monster in Round 1.

In Round 2, maybe the monster offers you gifts: superiority, ego, the ability to think fast. How nice! Then the monster just sits back and watches you beat yourself up by not sleeping, partying, gambling—ruining your life. When you are lying flat on your face and have had your car repossessed, been evicted from your apartment, been left by your significant other, and lost your job, you look around for the bearer of gifts, but he has abandoned you. He's probably back in his monster den, laughing about all the silly things you did.

Maybe in Round 1, you had to be admitted to a psych ward with all those "crazy" people. You were scared and resisted. The doctors put you on medication that made you feel operational, but not very "chirpy." After talking to the people in the psych ward, you found some who weren't so crazy. In Round 2, you weren't fond of the idea of going to the psych ward, but maybe your thoughts were racing so fast and you felt so suicidal and agitated that you would do anything to make the feelings go away. The psychiatrist and nurses had to help remove you from the clutches of the bipolar monster. You felt drained and exhausted afterward.

Maybe by Round 3, you learned to avoid the monster. The monster offers his gifts again, but you refuse. The monster tries to take away your common sense, bombarding you with racing thoughts so you can't seem to calm down enough to have a true thought of your own. By Round 3, you may be able to call your doctor and say, "Yo, Doc! Are there any beds available in the psych ward?"

You're learning. Maybe there won't be a Round 4—or maybe if there is, you will kick the monster's butt.

You see how it works?

Real People

One young woman reports that she ruined her life with mania, which she admitted being addicted to, three times. Three times she lost her apartment, car, boyfriend, and job. During the mania, she didn't care. She said she could always get a new apartment, a new car, a new boyfriend, and a new job. When she was 25, she had a long hypomanic episode and ended up with mononucleosis (from lack of sleep and a depressed immune system). She had a hard time recovering from the depression and chronic fatigue that followed. She decided that she didn't want to live her life that way, took her medication, and listened to the people who were trying to help her. At this writing, she is 34 years old and has been stable for nine years.

How Bipolar Changes with Age

Most scientists believe that the "kindling effect" will make untreated bipolar disorder worse. With a seizure disorder we know that the more seizures a person has, the more that person is likely to have. We have observed phenomenologically that the kindling effect makes a seizure disorder worse and that's why the doctors work so hard to prevent seizures. Most doctors believe the same thing is true for bipolar disorder: the more episodes a person has, the more that person is likely to have. Dr. Robert M. Post of the National Institute of Mental Health (NIMH) was the first to apply the kindling model to bipolar disorder. Doctors work hard to prevent episodes so that the patient does not develop rapid cycling and treatment-resistant bipolar disorder.

BP in General

The euphoric mania of bipolar disorder is most often seen in children and young adults. By middle age (between ages 40 and 60), mania seems to manifest mostly as agitation, anger, or apparent anxiety. If a person has been properly medicated in the previous years, she may be able to enjoy long periods of being symptom-free in middle age, or she may experience symptoms without full-blown episodes. If a person has been unmedicated or not properly medicated, however, middle age may be a period of rapid cycling and treatment resistance.

A 1999 study indicated that a high percentage of dual-diagnosis patients (substance abuse and bipolar) had a history of medication noncompliance, which would have accelerated the kindling effect. Substances such as cocaine and alcohol have their own kindling effects that can contribute to bipolar kindling. The realization that cocaine causes seizures led Dr. Post to connect kindling in epilepsy with mood disorders.

People who have been taking lithium compliantly for years show very little kindling effect, it seems. Those who have been on and off medication or who have had no medication at all have the most problems in middle age.

Let's look at an example of the adolescent who wakes up one morning feeling incredibly good. Is he motivated to seek treatment? Probably not. He may not realize that the mania directly corresponds to depression. As he matures, he may not get as much euphoric mania as anger, but even then, the ego, arrogance, and entitlement that go with the anger may feel good. As he approaches middle age and starts to have agitation (which he may experience as "anxiety"), he may go for help. The doctor may give him a benzodiazepine, which is not known to impede the kindling effect. It masks the symptoms, but the kindling effect may still be in process.

NAA is the second most-abundant amino acid (after glutamate) in the brain. Low NAA levels are an indication that the integrity of neurons or axons in the brain has been compromised, causing progressive brain damage. People who have had bipolar disorder the longest have the lowest levels of NAA. Research at the University of California shows that lithium has a protective effect on the brain. It has been shown to actually increase the amount of NAA and gray matter in the human brain.

The hippocampus plays an important role in bipolar disorder (influencing emotions and moods). Brain imaging has shown a smaller hippocampus in people with depression. The good news is that neuronal growth can occur in the hippocampus, possibly reversing damage.

Based upon the article "The Long-Term Natural History of the Weekly Symptomatic Status of Bipolar I Disorder" (*The Archives of General Psychiatry*, June 2002) and the feedback from more than 18,000 mental health professionals, along with having done more than 6,000 evaluations and having experienced bipolar disorder firsthand in my family, I have come up with four stages of bipolar disorder. I have given each of these stages an approximate age span. This model does not fit everyone who has bipolar disorder. It's just based upon the previous information and my own phenomenological observations. These examples are meant to demonstrate the type of person with bipolar disorder who is not likely to seek help, and therefore unlikely to prevent the kindling effect with medication. This is a person who likes the highs and may be addicted to the mania.

Euphoric Stage (Adolescence to Age 25)

The mania in this stage of bipolar disorder may be addicting. The person feels good. She thinks faster than others, doesn't seem to require as much sleep as others, and exhibits ego (which feels like self-esteem), arrogance (which feels like confidence), and entitlement (which may feel like a sense of purpose). This person is not going to get help. She feels too good. Others may even envy the way she's always enthusiastic and animated.

Of course, not all bipolar disorder starts out this way, and the age range may be slightly different. If a person does a lot of cocaine during this stage, for example, it may exacerbate the bipolar disorder and accelerate the kindling effect. This description does not include people who experienced agitation as a first indication of mania, and it does not include people who become psychotic and are hospitalized.

Angry Stage (Ages 25 to 40)

The mania in this stage is mostly anger (actually internal rage). The person has learned that the anger may intimidate people, so she uses it to her best advantage (in the same way that any human being uses a trait to his or her best advantage). She is angry, which may not seem like a lot of fun, but she also has ego, arrogance, and entitlement along with the anger, which may give her a sense of superiority. By this time, she has usually experienced the depths of depression, so the anger, at least, feels alive. She may not get help at this stage because "it's not so bad," and her bipolar disorder could be mistaken for something else—an anger management problem or personality disorder.

About 31 percent of people with bipolar disorder go more than 10 years before they are diagnosed. The person with this particular type of bipolar disorder is especially prone to being overlooked, because of the way her bipolar disorder emerges. It is a long time before she seeks help.

Rapid Cycling Stage (Ages 40 to 50)

Rapid cycling can occur at any age. Most children with BP are rapid cyclers. However, the rapid cycling in this stage is a result of the kindling effect. At this point, the bipolar disorder is getting worse. A person may ask for help at this stage because she feels "anxiety" (agitation). The doctor may give her a benzodiazepine, which masks the symptoms, but does not protect the brain's NAA. The kindling effect is not inhibited. The doctor may try to medicate for bipolar disorder, but if the patient is rapid cycling, she may experience large peaks and valleys and go off and on the medication. Rapid cyclers are difficult to medicate.

Schizoaffective Stage (End of Middle Age to Old Age)

At this stage, the person may fit the diagnostic criteria for schizoaffective disorder, but the symptoms are the result of the kindling effect of bipolar disorder. Schizoaffective disorder can be diagnosed when a person has delusions, hallucinations, disorganized speech, grossly disorganized behavior, and grossly inappropriate emotional responses. She becomes unable to form context, and her executive functions may stop working at times to such an extent that she appears to be incoherent. Other times, she may be normal and able to communicate appropriately.

The preceding are the four stages of kindling effect I made up to simplify the concept. Now that we have given one rendition of kindling effect, let's leave the "kindling effect" and take at look at the problems of the elderly and bipolar disorder.

BP in the Elderly

The symptoms of BP in younger children and older adults often appear similar. A number of studies suggest that the mixed emotional states and accelerated rapid cycling are alike. Mood swings and psychosis are common features of BP in children, as well as in older adults. Depression is likely the first prodromal sign in children and the elderly. The use of antidepressants in the elderly and children with bipolar disorder tends to speed up cycling and cause agitated depression.

Involutional depression may occur in elderly people who have BP. This is a traditional name for a psychiatric disorder affecting mostly elderly or late-middle-aged people, usually accompanied with paranoia. Again, people who have been stably medicated for bipolar disorder throughout their lives are less likely to experience this distress.

Causes of mania in the elderly:

◆ They are bipolar patients who are not currently medicated or are medicated improperly.

◆ Elderly patients with depression may develop manic-looking symptoms.

◆ Elderly patients may have organic brain diseases. Fifty percent have no past history of a mood disorder or have organic brain disease. Thirteen percent have had mania in the past. Thirty percent have a prodromal depression.

Elderly bipolar patients become unstable because of …

◆ Medication noncompliance due to loss of hope, death of caregiver, forgetfulness, or substance abuse.

◆ The kindling effect.

◆ Discontinuation of bipolar medication by the doctor because of organ deterioration.

Patients with dementia or delirium can appear manic. Psychoses, agitation, paranoia, sleep disturbance, and hostility are symptoms common to both delirium and BP. Patients discontinue medicine for multiple reasons:

◆ Noncompliance

◆ Death of caregiver and loss of support

◆ Physician discontinuation due to perceived complications from medications (30 percent renal failure may necessitate going off lithium)

Red Flag

Because of unstable insulin levels in the elderly, it is extremely important to monitor the effect of medications. The antipsychotics can cause insulin levels to become unstable and make an elderly person sick. Also take into account that elderly people's bodies do not process medication as quickly as younger people's do, and so elderly people may hold medication in the body longer. For these reasons, it is important to check sugar levels, liver enzymes, and the kidneys. Doctors and nurses are aware of these factors when treating the elderly.

The elderly living at home must have someone keep track of the medications they are on. Forgetfulness is typical among the elderly. It is also important that any medication interactions be monitored. If an elderly person has more than one doctor, it is absolutely essential that all the doctors know all the medications the person is taking. Make sure the pharmacy has a computer system that automatically assesses medication contraindications as a backup to avoid negative interactions. There are also websites available for you to check the medications yourself.

Real People

A physician diagnosed herself with bipolar disorder when she was 30 years old. She prescribed herself lithium and that stabilized her. She never told a soul about it, not even her spouse. She understood the stigma and quietly treated herself. She practiced medicine for 25 more years. Her patients thought the world of her and she was never involved in a malpractice suit. When she was 55 years old, she had to go to the hospital for a hysterectomy. Due to complications, she ended up in the ICU for a couple days, heavily medicated. When they took her off the medication, she became psychotically manic, which was attributed to a psychosis that some older people develop when recovering from anesthesia. But the psychotic mania was actually due to a sudden cessation of lithium.

The Least You Need to Know

♦ Although bipolar disorder can go into remission for years, when it does reappear, it can be subtle, and the signs needs to be made apparent.

♦ Take your medication. If you have had trouble taking your medication in the past, get someone to help, because the alternative could ruin your life.

♦ Approach bipolar disorder like a fighter. Each time you get knocked down in a round with the bipolar monster, you learn something to help defeat the monster and it may be easier to get back up.

16

Finding and Keeping a Job

In This Chapter

- ◆ Advice for bipolar job-seekers
- ◆ What to tell your employer and when
- ◆ How to ask for necessary accommodations

Bipolar disorder may affect all aspects of your life—including your job. In this chapter, we'll discuss how this condition can impact your role as an employee.

How Perceptions Have Changed

In yesteryear, employers took the good days and the bad days. A person could be productive for many years and then experience depression for a while and have his productivity drop. Twenty percent of our population has been depressed, and some of that depression is bipolar depression. Eventually the employee's depression would pass and the employee would become productive again.

But now employees are more likely to lose their jobs over diminished functioning. The companies have less invested in the well-being of their employees, and the employee has less flexibility to adapt to the workplace during episodes. Employees may work incapacitated and not inform their supervisors of their health issues, out of fear of losing their jobs. Yet hiring, firing, and job turnover are quite considerable expenses to employers. Chances are they will end up hiring someone else who was let go from their employer for diminished job performance due to depression. Have things gotten better for employers? It doesn't look that way. Things have also gotten worse for the good employee who is temporarily "down." We allow downtime and preventative maintenance for machines, but not for people.

It may not be fair, but knowing the way it is can be helpful in your negotiations at work. Maybe you would like to help your employer out by taking that midnight shift job, but your employer is not going to visit you in the psych ward after you have a manic episode. In fact, your employer may get rid of you for nonperformance a few weeks after you return to work, before you have time to recover from your ordeal and get your prefrontal lobe back online. So, no, don't take that midnight shift job. Don't work all that overtime, even if they need you "really bad," if it might wake up the bipolar monster. If your ego starts telling you that you can do these things, the bipolar monster may have already arrived and be about to pounce.

Many people with bipolar disorder have their own businesses and people that work for them. It's ideal, in a way. If you have a manic moment and tell off a customer, no one will fire you. If you just can't get out of bed one day, you can call and cancel an appointment. If you have at least one trusted employee with a consistent prefrontal lobe operating, that employee can take over for you during your down moments.

Things to Keep in Mind When Job Seeking

You may be worried that your bipolar disorder will be a big strike against you. It is your decision when and how to disclose it to a potential employer. Remember: you are not required to disclose mental health problems you have had in the past.

When looking for a job, try to find a position and/or line of work that will be the best possible fit for you and the requirements of your bipolar disorder. If, for example, you are more prone to problems when your sleep schedule is disrupted, avoid jobs where you work long hours or irregular shifts.

You might also want to look for companies with good benefits, especially health insurance coverage. If possible, try to find out about the specific mental health coverage offered by the company.

A job where you can optionally work at home would be ideal for those days when your emotions are amplified or you are not feeling up to interacting with people. Automobile travel is usually a good situation for people with BP. Driving can be soothing and there is usually an excuse to drive if you are having a bad day and need to get away.

Look for a tolerant atmosphere. If it looks like everyone is wound up tight and the boss is brash, you may have a manic moment, tell off the boss, and get fired. It is nice if you can make a mistake and apologize for it later. A tolerant atmosphere is an asset, bipolar or not.

It is helpful to sharpen your communication skills. Perhaps a Dale Carnegie course or an interpersonal communications course would be helpful. This is where your bipolar group therapy may be handy to bounce things off of and get good feedback. Be ready with the tools to repair relationships.

When looking for a job or applying for an available position, you want to make yourself look as good as possible. This includes grooming, mental acuity, and dress. Get someone to check you out before you go on the interview. Make sure you are "seeing yourself."

Protective Laws and Legal Documents

There are laws designed to protect employees with disabilities and special needs. Your best bet is to fly under the radar of any disability and not make it an issue. If it becomes an issue, there are certain rights you have as explained in the following sections.

Visible Disability

If a job candidate arrives at an interview with a Seeing Eye dog, an employer immediately recognizes that the candidate is legally blind. If the person is qualified and able to perform the tasks outlined in the job description, his blindness cannot be used as a reason to deny him the job. Right? Well … legally true, but not always the case.

It is legal for the employer to ask the blind candidate what, if any, accommodations, such as readers or other assistive technologies, will be needed for him to do his job. If an employer knows that she will have to make accommodations for a disabled person, she may be less likely to hire him, despite his suitability to a particular job. Expensive accommodations can cost the company money—and maybe the employer is allergic to dogs.

Despite the potential for tax breaks given to companies who hire disabled people and the grants available to cover the costs of assistive technologies, employers may decide to hire other similarly qualified individuals rather than be bothered with dogs and readers. It will be difficult, if not impossible, to prosecute the employer for discrimination if she does not explain her line of thinking to the applicant. Unfortunately, people with visible disabilities are often passed over for good job opportunities, but fortunately, people with invisible disabilities are often hired.

Invisible Disability

Bipolar disorder allows you a chance to prove yourself as a valuable employee before having to negotiate workplace accommodations.

If you suffer from bipolar disorder, you should be aware of laws that protect your rights. It is against U.S. federal law to ask a job candidate to submit to a medical examination so that the employer can know if the candidate has a disability before offering him or her a job. No one goes to a job interview with a sign on her chest stating that she is bipolar. It comes down to personal preference whether to disclose this disability to your employer.

Many people choose to keep their bipolar disorder a secret from their employers. Most people do not discuss their illness with their employers unless it interferes with their ability to perform their duties. This may seem unfair to the employer, who is left high and dry, so to speak, when you are unable to work. On the other hand, bipolar people realize that people, out of ignorance, are often biased against the mentally ill. As a result, they fear discrimination in spite of the many protections that federal and state laws provide. It is probably safer to wait until after an employer has gotten to know your qualifications and is satisfied with your performance to explain your deficits and special needs. With bipolar disorder, you may never have to explain as long as you can keep the bipolar monster at bay.

The Americans with Disabilities Act (ADA) formally recognizes severe mental illness as equal to physical illness. Both are disabilities. The ADA covers employers with 15 or more employees, including state and local governments. Under the ADA, all disabled persons have federal legal protection against discrimination by employers, landlords, and service providers.

Employers are required to afford you the same rights, privileges, and opportunities as they would persons with any other type of disability. Once you inform your employer of your disability, he or she must make reasonable accommodations that allow you to keep and perform your job, such as time off from work during an episode or for a hospitalization. It is understandable to choose to wait until you and your employer have begun a working relationship to disclose your disability. However, in the long run, it may be best to disclose your bipolar disorder and reach an understanding with your employer *before* you need to be accommodated for your illness. This decision is up to you and should be based upon the possibility of your disorder affecting your work. If you have had one episode when you were 18 and you have maintained a job and not had another for five years, the chances are that your employer will never have to know.

On the other hand, if you have always had problems every winter with bipolar depression, it is probably in your best interest to inform your employer that you may require some accommodations in the winter. Maybe you can work it out with your employer that you will take your personal days, sick days, and vacation days in the winter.

If you disclose your disability to your employer and you feel that reasonable accommodations are not being made or that you are being treated unfairly, several agencies can assist you. The U.S. Equal Employment Opportunity Commission (EEOC) enforces the employment provisions of the ADA and can help you with problems in the workplace. Additionally, every state has enacted laws for the Protection and Advocacy for Individuals with Mental Illness (PAIMI). PAIMI programs vary by state but are always fashioned to help people with mental illness deal with problem employers, landlords, and service providers. Often legal action against discriminating employers and others can be avoided by mediation with a PAIMI advocate. However, when necessary, PAIMI programs can provide free legal service on behalf of their mentally ill clients.

See Appendix B for the EEOC and PAIMI web addresses. Living with a severe mental illness like bipolar disorder, which is considered a medical disability, affords you well-deserved special protection under the law. Don't allow employers to illegally fire you or refuse to recognize the legitimacy of your disorder. It's the law!

If You Already Have a Job

Let's say you're already employed. Ideally, things are going well and you've had no problems. But, as you know, bipolar disorder is unpredictable, and you can never really be sure when you will experience symptoms. It's usually a good idea to be open and honest with your employer, so he or she won't be caught off-guard if you have a problem. Ask your supervisor if he or she knows anything about bipolar disorder. If not, bring in materials covering the information you want him or her to know. Decide with your boss if others should know. If you've already had an incident that everyone knows about, it is usually a good idea to explain it rather than leave it a mystery. You may also choose to talk about the symptoms of bipolar disorder (for example, "dyssomnia," or sleep disorders) without saying "bipolar disorder." The whole point in telling anyone is to make things easier on yourself, not more difficult. You can only give people what they are capable of understanding. They may not understand "bipolar," but probably would understand a sleep problem like "insomnia."

What to Tell Your Employer

If you feel that you need job accommodations, you may decide to tell your employer about your bipolar disorder. Ask yourself four questions: when, who, how, and what.

When do you tell anyone at work? You tell someone when you need accommodations. Perhaps you were out sick in the psych ward for a week. Perhaps you can't seem to think straight. Maybe you are having trouble with your medication. Maybe you just can't get out of bed in the morning.

Whom do you tell? You tell the person who can authorize the accommodation you need.

How do you tell this person? You can tell him that you have a medical condition. If you are looking for a more flexible starting time, you can tell him that you have a sleep dyssomnia. If you are having trouble thinking, you can tell him that you have a neurological problem from time to time. You could also tell him that you have bipolar disorder. Unfortunately, many people do not understand bipolar disorder and may stereotype you as someone who is liable to "go off." If you say "neurological problem" or "sleep dyssomnia," you're telling the truth without incurring the stereotypes or stigma.

What accommodations do you need? Here are some specific things you may want to ask for from your employer:

- A flexible schedule
- The ability to work from home
- A self-paced workload
- A part-time work schedule
- Uninterrupted work time
- Larger work assignments divided into smaller steps

- Daily "to do" lists

- Someone to prioritize the day's workload for you

- Positive reinforcement

- Sensitivity training for your supervisor or colleagues

- Flexible leave

- Periodic meetings to discuss work productivity and workplace issues

You may need any of the preceding temporarily. If you just had an episode and your thinking is not clear, your ability to think straight will come back as soon as your prefrontal lobe is online again. You may need a part-time work schedule if you are trying to get through a particularly tough depression. You may need flexible leave to attend an outpatient program. You may need someone to give you a daily "to do" list, prioritize your workload, or break down large tasks into smaller tasks.

You may also need some of these items on a permanent basis. Maybe mornings are always difficult for you. Perhaps your employer can put you on an adapted work schedule from 11:00 A.M. to 7:00 P.M., for example, or on second shift from 3:00 P.M. to 11:00 P.M. (No midnight shifts, please.) Perhaps you can come in late every day and make it up by working part of Saturday.

The best scenario is to be able to accommodate yourself without inconveniencing your employer. If you do inconvenience your employer, perhaps you can make it up in other ways. You want to remain a valuable employee while keeping your sanity at the same time.

Mental Note

Under the Americans with Disabilities Act, a person with a disability is not required to disclose it unless seeking an accommodation at work.

Real People

In one division of a large corporation, most people came in to work at 7:00 A.M. and left at 3:30 P.M. Most people liked this schedule because they were able to avoid heavy traffic before and after work. One man came in at 10:00 A.M. and left at 6:30 P.M., and there was talk about how he came in "late" every day. Someone said something to his manager, who said, "Well, he stays until 6:30 or later. I can arrange your schedule that way, too, if you wish!" The employee sheepishly said, "No, thanks." The man got more respect after that.

You may want to keep the reason for your accommodation between you and your supervisor. You may also want to discuss how your boss is going to explain it to others. Most bosses are fairly good about this and may say to an inquisitor, "I asked him to come in these hours and work Saturday. Are you interested in working Saturday, too?"

Of the 54 mental disability cases brought to trial in 2004, 41 resulted in employer wins, 13 were unresolved, and none favored the employee. Eight cases involved people with substance disorders. Of these, six resulted in employer wins, two were not resolved, and none favored the employee. The good news is that employers do not want the overhead and stigma of going to court over these issues and may settle an issue to avoid the hassle.

Communicating with Coworkers

Employees with mental health problems may experience stigma and discrimination from coworkers if their mental illnesses become known. Workers who return from bouts of mental illness report returning to positions of reduced responsibility and increased supervision. They may become targets for mean-spirited or negative comments from coworkers who were previously friendly. About half of the people with a serious mental illness who have a competitive job are eventually terminated as a result of interpersonal problems.

In order to avoid workplace stigma and discrimination, employees with mental health problems often go to great lengths to ensure that their coworkers do not find out. They may avoid EAPs (employee assistance programs) and pay for treatment out of pocket instead of using their employer-provided health-care benefits.

Research shows that people who are bullies in school often have the same mental health problems as their victims. If you have a mental health problem, you may have just reminded a bully of his greatest fear. If the bully makes you the scapegoat, he thinks, maybe no one will notice his own problems. Most bullies have big egos to hide their poor self-esteem. One solution for this type of behavior is to get the bully alone, without his audience. Just look him straight in the eye and politely tell him that you don't appreciate him embarrassing you or putting you down.

If it does get out that you are the company "nut case," just admit it with a sense of humor. Say something profound like, "I may be nuts, but I'm not stupid." Anything you can confront, you can handle. Go out of your way to repair relationships. It's not your fault that your coworkers doubt you, but you may have to take responsibility to assuage their doubts. There is a big difference between responsibility and blame.

Real People

A woman who was president of a large, prestigious association was scheduled to give a speech at their annual convention. A month before the convention, she had had a manic episode, during which she pushed a police officer, and she had been incarcerated for a couple weeks. She knew that some of the 200 association members attending the speech knew she had been in jail. She was terrified to make the speech, to the point of a near anxiety attack. She was advised by a close friend to talk about her incarceration and get it out of the way instead of trying to hide it.

When she took the podium, everyone was unusually quiet. She started her speech: "How are y'all doing this evening? I am proud to say that I am probably the first president of this association to go to jail." Some laughter came from the crowd, and some exclamations of surprise. "And they say there's no such thing as a free lunch! I am here to tell you that I had two weeks of free lunches, free medical care, and the company of 1,200 innocent people."

The crowd roared; her addressing the matter relieved everyone's anxiety. After the laughter died down, she said, "Now that I am all rested up, let's talk about our goals for this coming year …."

Humor is one of the best ways to release tension. Exaggerating what people are thinking is humorous and acknowledges their feelings. As soon as you acknowledge people's feelings, they can move on; otherwise, they stay stuck in the present, unexpressed feeling. For example, when you show up for a meeting after a trip to the psych ward, your coworkers may all stare at you uncomfortably. What do you say? If you wanted to exaggerate the situation, you might smile and say, "Did you save a seat for the crazy guy?"

Once everyone knows you were in the psych ward, you have nothing to lose. Ham it up. Read joke books about mental health. Bipolar disorder is a physiological illness that makes people *act* crazy, but *they are not crazy*. If you are approachable and open about your disease, you will have a chance to educate your coworkers and get them on your side.

Do your work and do it as well as you can. If you can't, tell your coworkers that your brain cells are temporarily off-line, but that your doctor says they will be back in a few weeks. Separate your work performance from your mental disorder. These are two separate issues.

People with bipolar disorder can sometimes miss social cues. As we have said before, the actions of people with BP who are a bit symptomatic can be misinterpreted. Being specific and direct can be helpful at these times. This usually happens when the pre-frontal lobe is out or partially out and the person with BP doesn't see the bigger picture or context. People with BP can be very concrete or literal at times, and they may not understand jokes or certain insinuations.

Real People

A boss with BP was at work with his employees at 2:00 on Christmas Eve. The three other bosses had let their people go at 1:00. As the boss walked by, one of his employees said, "Gee. Nobody is here except us." Preoccupied by his racing thoughts, the boss said, "Yeah," and kept walking. He was a good boss and normally very accommodating. His employees started talking among themselves:

"Maybe he is angry with us for something."

"Maybe he is so cheap, he wants us to work."

"Maybe he is bah-humbug about Christmas."

Finally, one employee went down to the boss's office and said, "Hey, Boss! Can we leave early, since it's Christmas and we have some last-minute shopping?"

"Oh, sure," the boss said, and he went down to tell everyone to go home.

If Problems Arise

Recent research shows that support from employers for equity and workplace accommodations has been low. Compliance with legislative requirements has not been entirely forthcoming. In the United States, mental disorders are the second most-common basis for charges of discrimination and workplace harassment under the Americans with Disabilities Act.

Larger corporations, which have written policies for managers to follow, usually have better compliance. And most companies would rather make some sort of settlement than risk a court case. If you are under treatment for your bipolar disorder and your company will grant you a severance package and continue your insurance, that may be exactly what you need until you can recover enough to take another job. The chances that your company will release confidential information about your mental illness are slim to none. Once you are stable and able to work again, you are less likely to run into the same problems. Again, each time the bipolar monster throws a banana peel in your path, you learn to dodge it a little better.

If there are gaps in your employment, you may want to explain them in some plausible way. You could just simply say, "I just needed some time off." That is a call you will have to make for yourself. Unfortunately, telling a potential employer that you have bipolar disorder and that, though you may have an episode now and then, you are a really good employee, may not have positive results.

The secret to maintaining full employment is to set your life up so that you interrupt each episode that you might otherwise have. The bipolar monster doesn't get frustrated, he just goes away. He is what he is. Nothing personal.

> **Research Says**
>
> Bipolar disorder is the sixth leading cause of disability in the world, according to the World Health Organization. Depression is one of the leading causes of sick leave and may soon be the leading cause of absenteeism in the workplace.

When it comes to problems that you don't want people to know about, it is all right to lie to people for whom your health is none of their business or who would never understand anyway. Maybe someday bipolar disorder will be as widely accepted as diabetes, with no stigma attached, but that day is not here yet. But public awareness is increasing. Bipolar disorder is in the news and on Oprah. Some pretty high-powered, successful people have come out of the bipolar closet. Things are looking up.

Real People _____

Dr. Kay Jamison and other psychologists note the propensity for the positive emotions to be overlooked by psychologists and psychiatrists. She notes that exuberance, enthusiasm, purpose, and passion for life can override depression and become more important than the depression. The passion for her work overrides her bipolar disorder.

Managing Someone with BP

The information in this section can be applied to general management of a person with BP (for example, a son or daughter) as well as in a work relationship. This author worked in management at IBM and found people with BP easy to manage. Here's what I noticed about the people with BP who worked for me:

- They love to keep busy.

- They have great outside-of-the-box ideas.

- They can get obsessed with a project and hyperfocused to the point where it gets done in record time.

- They may do exactly what you say in the order you say it.

- You shouldn't take their mood swings personally.

- You can usually switch a mood swing easily with a joke or encouragement.

- Never directly criticize someone with BP. Instead, tell him or her, "It might be better if …."

- If they get annoyed with people and distracted, give them a quiet empty office and allow them to close the door and focus on their work.

- If they have trouble with their prefrontal lobe one day, help them prioritize their work and be specific about the tasks, putting them in writing. It doesn't take long.

- If they get too many good ideas and can't stop talking, give them a task to do.

Most of the time, a person with bipolar disorder performs normally, and when he or she does not, these management techniques take very little effort and often reap excellent results. If you think that an employee may not be taking her medication, you may have to have a talk with her. You may have to become her temporary prefrontal lobe and reiterate the bigger picture in a nonthreatening way. Explain that you have noticed that her duties fall behind when she is not taking her medication. You cannot make her take her medication, but it is your job as her manager to monitor her work-load and give feedback.

If you are managing or supervising someone with bipolar disorder, you may run into problems here and there that are surmountable with the right understanding. I have heard many bosses say that an employee with BP was "a heck of a good worker, but …"

Here are some of the buts:

"He told me off in front of the other workers, and I can't have that kind of disrespect."

"She calls in sick all the time."

"He is late every day."

"She says inappropriate things to other people."

"He says rude things to others and antagonizes them."

For most people with bipolar disorder, these things happen temporarily, during symptomatic periods. There are several things a manager can easily do to fix the problem. Ask the person into your office to talk. Try to pick a time when he or she is not agitated, and be friendly and personable.

For example: "I really like you, Ben. I really admire your work and how much you get done in one day, but it looks like you're having some difficulty right now."

Ask him if he minds if you ask a few questions. If he says okay, remind him that you know he has bipolar disorder. Is he taking his medication? Is he getting enough sleep? Is something stressing him out?

Advise the person that it may be time to address the issue before it gets out of hand. Sometimes it is appropriate to just tell a person's coworkers, individually or as a group, that the person is having a hard time at the moment and not to take his behavior personally. If you think it would be best to say something to the person's coworkers, discuss with him how that should be done: "Should we tell them you have something like Tourette's syndrome and can't help saying things that may upset them? Should we tell them you have bipolar disorder and explain it? Should I have a meeting with everyone? Should I meet with certain individuals? Do you want to be present at the meeting? Do you want to say something to them yourself?"

Assure the person that you don't want to lose him (if he is a good worker) and that you will work with him to solve any problems. State the current problem in a non-threatening way. Just state the facts without criticism, judgment, or a raised voice. Come up with a solution between you and be specific about it, possibly writing it down: "Do you need a different start time? Do you need to see your doctor? Do you need me to call you to make sure you are up?"

Many times, employers lose good people because the employee has a manic moment or because of bipolar symptoms that can be easily accommodated. It doesn't take long to understand BP from a workplace standpoint, and it doesn't take long to manage it in an employee when it comes up. Bipolar symptoms are usually a temporary condition that will pass, and you will have a grateful, productive employee in the long run. Again, the main problems you will see are ...

- Symptoms from not remembering to take medication.

- Manic moments.

- Temporary substance abuse residuals (hangover).

- Lateness.

In conclusion, let me say I have not had to stay on top of these problems. They have been temporary spikes in an otherwise productive working relationship. I have more problems with employees who don't know they have problems.

The Least You Need to Know

- ◆ Choosing your job and employer carefully can help lessen the chances of problems on the job.

- ◆ When requesting accommodations, ask only for things you really need. Otherwise, it will look like you're just using your condition as a way to get nice perks.

- ◆ If you establish yourself as a valuable employee, your boss will be more likely to accommodate your special needs.

- ◆ The best intervention is prevention.

- ◆ Don't lose a good employee for a problem that is easily fixed.

Chapter 17

Family and Social Life

In This Chapter

- ◆ The secret to relationships
- ◆ Helping others help you
- ◆ How BP affects sexuality
- ◆ Hypersexuality versus sexual addiction
- ◆ The universal intervention

Bipolar disorder doesn't just affect the person who has the disorder. It also affects that person's friends, family, and coworkers—and just about anyone who interacts with the bipolar person on a regular basis.

In this chapter, we'll describe the ways that bipolar disorder affects the people around you. We will also discuss ways you can minimize any damage to your relationships as a result of BP.

BP and Relationships

A relationship involves two people, both of whom must make an effort to keep the relationship going. If one person is temporarily incapable of perceiving contexts, he is incapable, for that time, of perceiving relationships.

Such is the dilemma with people in relationships with people who have bipolar disorder. No prefrontal lobe working? No relationship perceived.

Sometimes there are things we might like to say to our spouse, but we don't because we can weigh the consequences on the relationship. If your prefrontal lobe is not working, however, you cannot perceive context, and therefore cannot perceive relationship. Relationships are contexts. You have no executive functions available to weigh things. If you are agitated and your brain is temporarily connected directly to your tongue, you are probably going to create a relationship problem, however unwittingly.

In previous chapters, we have shown how people in a manic state don't have the ability to see themselves or put themselves in someone else's place. This happens in various degrees, but the bottom line is that when this occurs, the person with BP can't help it. That is half of the problem. The other half is that the person the bipolar person affects may take whatever happens personally. It's important that the people around you know not to take these things personally. That might not be easy, so be prepared for some hurt feelings.

An Example

Once, a couple years ago, I had been giving seminars for a week, driving from one city to another. I had lost some sleep and it was finally Friday, my last day of work before flying home. At my last seminar, one man kept asking lengthy questions that required complicated, scientific knowledge. Luckily, I had answers, but by the third question, I realized that he already knew the answers and was trying to trip me up. One part of me got angry and was thinking, "He is disturbing the seminar and ticking me off. If he's going to be disruptive, I am going to verbally kick his butt."

However, the more enlightened part of me walked over to him (standing over him for a little dominance) and said, smiling in a personable manner, "Do I remind you of anyone?"

He thought for a moment and then smiled. "Yes," he said, "You remind me of my uncle."

I said, "Did you like your uncle?"

He laughed and said, "No, I hated him. He was a year older than me and a know-it-all."

I said, "Do you have any more questions for me?"

Still laughing, he said, "No. I think I get it."

If I had taken his questioning personally, I might have caused a battle that would have made everyone uncomfortable. My seminar went on peacefully because I didn't take the disruption personally. It still affected me, and I still had to deal with it, but we deal with things much more constructively if we don't take them personally.

What "Not Taking Things Personally" Really Means

Some people think that "not taking it personally" means ignoring a person and discounting everything the person says. No! You still have to connect with and listen to the person, but listen past the antagonistic part.

I had a wealthy client with whom I had a good relationship. Whenever one of his brothers or sisters had a problem, he would send him or her to me. Eventually, I had seen all nine brothers and sisters. Out of the blue one day, the mother called me. She said, "I know my kids have all talked to you and I want to come in to set the story straight. I know they said some things about me."

She came in and was very upset. I let her go on for a while and then I said, "You know, kids blame their parents for everything. You had nine children. I am sure they haven't thought about how difficult that was. You can't take everything they say personally."

"What should I do?" she asked. "I don't remember half the things they accuse me of."

I said, "First, don't take it personally. Second, you might say something like, 'Did I do that? If I did that, I am sorry.'"

Some time later she called me and said, "It worked. When I said that, it stopped them in their tracks. Some of my girls started to cry then and told me they loved me. Wow!"

Everyone has their own perceptions, some of which only last a moment. When I was raising my bipolar child, I had to determine whether things she said to me came from the bipolar disorder or whether they were deliberately disrespectful. If she was manic, I wouldn't take what she said personally (no matter how cutting or how true her statements were). I also wouldn't mete out consequences for her statements; she couldn't help it if her brain was temporarily connected directly to her tongue. If I determined that her statements came from disrespect and I didn't see any bipolar stuff, there would be consequences. As a father, that was part of my job. But I still wouldn't take it personally. That doesn't mean I was a stoic computer. I would tell her how she hurt my feelings and that she needed to ask herself how her actions affected other people.

When you learn not to take things personally, it doesn't mean that you disassociate or disregard what the person says. It doesn't mean that you don't alter your behavior if you are wrong. You simply know that a person who thinks "it's all about me" does not function as well as someone who knows it isn't. This won't just benefit your bipolar loved one. It will benefit *you*.

The Importance of Socialization

Socialization is important for all human beings. We need regular contact with other people to be emotionally fulfilled and to develop healthy relationships. Bipolar people are no different. In fact, if anything, they need social contact more than most people, because they need the support and caring of the largest possible support system.

Red Flag

Socializing doesn't necessarily have to include things like bars and dance clubs. In fact, those places can often spell trouble for someone who is bipolar. It's probably a smart idea to bypass the clubs and instead stick to safer social activities (sports, volunteer work, meeting friends for coffee or lunch, and so on).

The problem, of course, is that bipolar people may not always feel like socializing—especially when they are depressed and just want to hide in their rooms alone. Yet this is exactly when they need social interaction the most. When you begin to feel depressed, the support of friends and family can help keep you from falling deeper into that pit. Maintaining a busy social life can also keep you too occupied to obsess over your problems or become more depressed.

It can be helpful if some of the people in your social circle are also bipolar, so they will understand what you're going through and are less likely to be thrown for a loop by your moods or other BP symptoms.

Help Others Help You

If you are bipolar, your loved ones probably really want to help you, but they don't know exactly how. Don't expect them to be mind readers. Let them know exactly what you need and how they can help. Since you may not be thinking clearly or communicating well during a manic phase or depressed period, it's a good idea to have a long talk with loved ones beforehand, when you're in a stable state of mind. If they are well-prepared and know what they should do during your bipolar episode, they'll feel more confident about their ability to help.

Here are some other things you can do to help your loved ones help you:

- ◆ **Educate them.** Share books, magazines, and online resources related to BP.

- ◆ **Inform them.** Tell them the most important things they can do, and when.

- ◆ **Include them.** Ask loved ones to join you in family therapy or support group meetings.

Bipolar and Your Sex Life

Bipolar disorder affects all of your relationships, including those of a sexual nature. In fact, BP can often cause some specific—and challenging—problems that can negatively impact your sex life in a major way.

Bipolar Hypersexuality

Hypersexuality is a big problem for some BP people. You may assume that the term simply means the need for a lot of sex—and you may wonder what's so terrible about that. In reality, though, this need usually leads to destructive sex, which can lead to serious negative consequences.

Hypersexuality combined with impaired judgment can ruin a bipolar person's marriage. Sexually transmitted diseases abound in this day and age, so hypersexuality can be deadly.

Not all people with bipolar disorder experience hypersexuality, but for those who do, it can be a serious problem. There are two essential recommendations:

def•i•ni•tion

Hypersexuality is an increased need, or even pressure, for sexual gratification. It is often a symptom of mania. In mania, it includes decreased inhibitions.

- ◆ Finding the right combination of bipolar medications

- ◆ Finding a support group, such as an SLAA (Sex and Love Addicts Anonymous) group

What is it like to be hypersexual? Recall your adolescence, when you had trouble controlling your sexual urges, and then multiply that by 10. Of course, in bipolar disorder, hypersexuality can be accompanied by other symptoms. Angst may be present in the form of agitation. An emptiness may be present that cannot seem to be filled. In some cases, acting out sexually can propel a person into a full-blown manic episode with obsessive thoughts, severe lack of sleep, and eventually psychotic behavior.

Red Flag

There have been many ruined marriages, unwanted pregnancies, and sexually transmitted diseases as a result of bipolar hypersexuality. Hypersexuality often gets over-looked as a symptom and the person who acts out is frequently misunderstood and treated badly—even by herself.

Hypersexuality is often not a moral issue, but a symptom of bipolar disorder. One must know how a person acts when he is not manic to know about his true personality and true morals. In desperation or lack of conscience (no prefrontal lobe online), people may act out sexually, only to have their morals come crashing down on them when the prefrontal lobe and the bigger picture come back. People may end up trying to resolve their cognitive dissonance—the gap between what they have done and their true morals—by justifying what they did or blocking out the memory. They may be in such conflict that they seriously contemplate suicide.

Sexual Addiction

Someone who has bipolar disorder may get desperate enough to start using illegal drugs to stop the angst. In the process, he may get addicted to the drug. The same thing is true of sexual addiction. It's not about the drug, it's about the mentality that develops. One starts rationalizing that as long as no one gets hurt, it's okay. As long as no one knows, it won't be an issue. There is not enough prefrontal lobe present to realize that if someone does find out, it will be the end of the marriage, misery for the children, and so on. The addict may rationalize about who is responsible, as in, "Well, if she were more loving and paid more attention to me, I wouldn't have to do this." If that is truly the case, then why not haul the marriage into counseling for a rehabilitation?

Mental Note

Looking back, some bipolar people with sex addictions may realize that their sex addiction traits developed early in life, even before their bipolar traits did. These people have two separate disorders, even though their symptoms may mix.

One characteristic of any addiction is to blame some-one, or some group, or society as a whole, or to come up with a crazy philosophy of why it's okay to con-tinue the addiction. That's one way you can tell it's an addiction: when the addict thinks she is continu-ing her behavior for a reason. I have heard most of the excuses; some of them are very creative and some even sound true.

With bipolar hypersexuality, the treatment is physiological. The right medication reduces the mania and the hypersexuality. If you have a sex addiction as well, it's time to see a sexual addictions counselor. In either case, I think it's a good idea to attend SLAA meetings. They are free and very informative, and you'll need them the next time the hypersexual bipolar monster awakens.

Insights from Mavis Humes

Sex addiction is not just liking sex. Sex addiction is becoming obsessed with particular aspects of sex, such as affairs, pornography, types of sex acts, or fantasies to the point where it is causing problems and interfering with your finances, relationships, health, safety, and functioning at work or school.

Many times, people with bipolar disorder report acting out sexually in a way that is not in their best interest due to a manic episode, and there is some confusion about the difference. People with bipolar disorder can also be sex addicts, or they can just be people having a manic or hypomanic episode and meanwhile acting out impulsively in several ways, including sexually. By contrast, sex addicts have a particular progressive and obsessive *pattern* of acting out sexually, to the point that it affects their thinking and their lifestyle.

I have been treating addictions and working with thousands of wonderful patients for over 20 years. You may suppose that a person with bipolar disorder does have a slightly greater risk for developing a sex addiction, and my professional observations confirm that. Yet, we see the majority of bipolar cases as not having an actual sex addiction, and we see the majority of sex addicts as not having bipolar disorder. One psychiatric review (Spaltz, 1974) found that personality disorder and alcohol and drug use were more associated with hypersexuality than was bipolar disorder. The biggest risk factors for sex addiction that have been identified so far (Carnes & Laaser, 1996) are coming from a rigid, disengaged family system and having suffered physical, emotional, and/or sexual abuse in childhood.

It seems that people with other mental health diagnoses in general are highly represented among those who become sex addicts. It is rare to have a sexually addicted client who does not have some other co-occurring diagnosis as well. We commonly see other addictions, mood disorders, depression, post-traumatic stress disorder, dissociative identity disorder, attention deficit disorder, personality disorders, and more.

If you are suffering from the negative consequences of compulsive sexual behavior, yet cannot stop or stay stopped, you will find real recovery in any of the 12-step programs that treat sex addiction, no matter what original causes you ascribe to your sex problems. The amazing thing about these programs, whether we like to admit it or not, is that they are specifically designed to treat sex addiction, and *they work!* When the person does the work and keeps at it, 12-step programs are life-changing and transformative, even for the most hopeless cases.

You can find a therapist who specializes in treating sex addiction to help you determine whether you need to treat your compulsive sexual behavior separately from your bipolar illness. You can find certified professionals through one of the websites that lists certified sex addiction therapists, such as www.iitap.com.

If you are thinking of leaving this determination up to your regular doctor or psychiatrist, please be careful! Most medical personnel are not trained to recognize or treat addictive disorders, and many of them do not even "believe" in them! You are also at greater risk of being misdiagnosed either as a sex addict or as not a sex addict, based on the bias of an inadequately trained clinician. However, clinicians who work specifically in the addictions field find it relatively simple to make these diagnoses correctly. It can be especially confusing for a person with bipolar disorder to recognize if he or she has a sex addiction or not, so if the resistance to 12-step recovery is very great, consulting with a professional who is specially trained to treat both sex addiction and bipolar disorder is usually necessary.

If you are concerned that you may have a sex or romance addiction, a good place to start is by taking the questionnaire published by one of the 12-step organizations for recovery from sex addiction, such as Sex Addicts Anonymous or Sex and Love Addicts Anonymous, to see if you identify with them. Those questionnaires were created by people who themselves are in recovery from sex addiction.

Nurturing—An Intervention

Do you want a really good intervention for bipolar disorder? This is the second best one. It's called nurturing. When someone is manic, don't bother to argue with him, get angry at him, or threaten him. None of that will work. Nurture him. You are *not* rewarding him, rather you are helping the person through a tough phase.

The Universal Intervention

According to a statistic, 50 percent of manic people admitted to a facility commit a violent act—that would be spitting, pushing, punching, stabbing, or shooting. Now, is that a statistic about people with BP, or is that a statistic about us? Do we know so little about mania that we provoke manic people into a violent act 50 percent of the time? I'll let you decide.

Between working at a rehab for six years and a jail for three years, I have been in a room alone with a person who is manic over 1,000 times and I have *never* had a manic person commit a violent act on me. Was I just really lucky? No, I just developed the universal intervention, which is the best intervention for almost any situation, including BP. It's a little difficult to explain, but it works.

No matter where you go and no matter what the situation, the secret to managing the situation is: affinity, acknowledgment, and admiration.

Affinity is doing something physical with a person, like shaking hands. This is the therapist who puts her hand on your arm as you are leaving her office. This is the spouse who gets up from the dinner table for a glass of water and makes sure she touches her husband on the shoulder with her hand as she passes by.

You have to show affinity in your own way. I cannot tell you how to do it; it has to fit your personality. Some people are extroverted and might give a person a big hug when greeting them. Others merely shake hands and smile. Some show they like you by giving you a slightly longer smile and looking into your eyes a little longer than usual, but not long enough to be intimidating.

Acknowledgement doesn't mean "agreement." You say, "Wow, now I see why you are upset." You acknowledge their feelings.

Admiration is the most valued concept besides love. It must be genuine. It's hard, sometimes, to be genuine. What do you admire about a drug dealer? "Hey, I like your gold chain." If you can't be genuine, then fake it until you make it.

When you are implementing the universal intervention, you are going to be too busy to think about your own insecurities because you are paying attention to what's outside yourself. Your motivation is going to be to connect with a person, acknowledge this person, and find something to admire about this person.

Practice this process. Greet a stranger (a smile equals affinity), say hello (acknowledge her existence), and find something to admire about her.

Once you are reasonably successful at developing the process in yourself, you might consider making this a strategy in your life. Once you make something a strategy, the behavior, feelings, and thoughts automatically follow. It becomes part of who you are. If you make something a goal, you may or may not reach the goal. If you make something a strategy, there can be an unlimited number of goals associated with it. You will come up with goal after goal, plan after plan.

The universal intervention does as much for you as it does for others. I didn't invent it; I just discovered it. I hope you do, too.

The Least You Need to Know

- ◆ Bipolar disorder doesn't just affect you. It also affects your family and friends.

- ◆ BP can be very stressful on relationships, but there are things you can do to minimize the challenge.

- ◆ Loved ones are probably eager to help you, but may not know how.

- ◆ BP can cause hypersexuality and sex addiction.

- ◆ Learn and practice the universal intervention.

Pregnancy and Bipolar Disorder

In This Chapter

◆ Bipolar's effect on pregnancy

◆ BP and breastfeeding

◆ The importance of planning your pregnancy

◆ Firsthand advice about bipolar pregnancy

◆ Bipolar treatments while pregnant

There is not a lot of research available about pregnancy. It is unethical to do double-blind studies on pregnant mothers, so we have to collect information from past single cases, one by one, and put it all together to come up with some probabilities. Luckily, some people have done that with the drugs that have been around for a while. The newer drugs have not been around long enough to measure the outcomes as far as birth defects and treatment effectiveness.

We are going to give you the information that people have collected, as well as feedback from Dr. Carter's seminar attendees who have treated pregnant women with BP over the last seven years. We highly recommend that you get the most up-to-date information from the NIMH, NAMI, and DBSA websites along with reading this chapter. New research is available all the time and (hopefully) this chapter will be outdated soon by this new research. As we have said before, you must not take this chapter as a personal recommendation. Always check with your doctor (psychiatrist, geneticist, obstetrician, nurse practitioner) before using any of the treatment options that may be suggested in this book.

The Issues of Pregnancy

Women who have bipolar disorder have some special issues surrounding pregnancy.

- ◆ Should I go off my medication?

- ◆ If I do, what are the chances I will have an episode?

- ◆ If I don't, what are the chances that if I continue my medication, will it affect my unborn child?

> **Research Says**
>
> Pregnant mothers with BP have twice the risk for an episode as women who have BP and are not pregnant. There is also a seven times greater chance of being admitted to a hospital for their BP. A study from the *American Journal of Psychiatry* found that pregnant women with BP who go off their medication during pregnancy have a high risk of having an episode.

The statistics stated in the margin note are from blanket research appearing in the *American Journal of Psychiatry*. It does not differentiate between planned and unplanned pregnancy, nor the environmental stability of the participants. The feedback (consensus) from mothers who had a planned pregnancy and had a stable environment was that they felt good during their pregnancy without medication. Although hormones and bipolar disorder are usually a difficult combination, it seems like Mother Nature helps out with bipolar women who are in a stable environment. Most of these women report (and so does the spouse) that there seems to be an added stability even after pregnancy.

One doctor treats environmentally stable pregnant women with BP by prescribing haloperidal PRN as needed. Most stable women end up not needing to take it, but if they can't sleep to the point that they may have an episode, a woman can safely take haloperidal which has been classified as "insignificant" for causing birth defects.

There are more statistics. These are not to alarm you, just to advise you. Women who suddenly stop their medication (pregnant or not) are more likely to have bipolar symptoms. We know this from observation (phenomenologically). Women who discontinue meds from six months before pregnancy to 12 weeks into pregnancy are twice as likely to have an episode. Women who discontinue meds experienced symptoms during almost half of their pregnancy, while those who continued meds experienced symptoms less than 10 percent of the time.

Planned Pregnancies

Obviously, this is the way to go, if you can. Gather up all the information you can, talk to your doctor (obstetrician, psychiatrist), and do this before conception. This will give you the best advantage to prevent episodes, birth defects, and family discord. In the United States, there is only an 8 percent chance of having a bipolar child if one parent has bipolar disorder. Get all this settled before the child is even a glint in Mama's eye.

The medications rated the best for being "insignificant" for causing birth defects are first generation medications (haloperidal and thorazine). They have been around long enough to be measured. Lithium has also been around for a long time. When lithium is used in the first trimester, there may be cardiac problems with the baby after the baby is born. The overall risk for anomalies is 4 to 12 percent (as shown by several studies). Lithium is much safer in the second and third trimester. If Mom decides to nurse the baby while on lithium, the baby should be checked for lithium blood levels.

Valproic acid has also been studied and shows an overall high risk for birth defects when taking 1,000 mg or more daily. It is determined to be safe in the eighth and ninth month, according to feedback. Vitamin K is recommended for mothers who are taking valproic acid. Tegretol is not recommended during pregnancy. Lamotrigne shows a small risk (if any) of birth defects for any major anomalies. The birth defect research of the other newer medications is not confirmed. Preliminary information from early studies indicate that olanzapine does not cause birth defects, but it has been associated with weight gain and diabetes. Weight gain and diabetes are significant concerns for the birth mother. An assessment for birth defects is significant because it may affect your child for a lifetime.

As more research is done, more information will be available on the effects of medication on the unborn child. It is recommended that expecting women take only one bipolar medication, as it is less harmful to the fetus than two or more. The dosages should be divided up throughout the day instead of taken all at once. If a woman is on lithium during pregnancy, she should keep herself hydrated (even more trips to the bathroom!) and the infant should be checked for lithium levels right after birth. If lithium is continued after birth, it reduces the possibility of bipolar symptoms to 10 percent.

Breast Feeding

Lithium (and most other drugs) get passed along with breast milk to the baby. If a woman insists on breast feeding while on lithium, the infant's blood levels should be checked for lithium.

Red Flag

Any psychotropic medication taken by the mother will be transmitted through the breast milk. The safest thing for Mom may be to go back on her medication as soon as the baby is born. This leaves the baby to be bottle fed, which can be done by Dad, Grandma, Grandpa, or another relative.

The American Academy of Pediatrics and the American Academy of Neurology indicate that valproic acid is safe for breast feeding.

Tegretol was found in low concentrations in breast milk and is also acceptable by the two aforementioned organizations. However, tegretol is *not* recommended *during* pregnancy due to complications and birth defects.

The first generation drugs (haliperdal and thorozine) appear to be safe during pregnancy and breast feeding.

Other Treatment

Electroconvulsive therapy (ECT) has fewer risks for the fetus than any of the medications. The heart rate and oxygen levels of the fetus can be monitored during ECT, which would detect any problems. Pregnant women who utilize ECT should make sure they are hydrated and have the proper diet and vitamins. In these cases, there is little probability of premature contractions.

Psychotherapy has been shown to improve the general day-to-day functioning of pregnant women.

Exercise (not manic overexertion) is helpful during pregnancy. Relaxation techniques and yoga seem to have great benefit. Massage is relaxing. Be sure to go to a therapeutic massage therapist who has been educated in the proper techniques for pregnant women. There are certain points of the body that should be avoided in massage so as not to cause contractions.

Sleep, as we said, is perhaps the most important part of maintaining stability in all cases. A woman may be pregnant with BP and be missing sleep to the point where she is getting run down, or is unable to sleep at all. It may be time to ask the doctor for some haloperidal, and ask loved ones for assistance in the judgment of taking medication for sleep. After one loses enough sleep, objectivity is an issue and Mom may need to borrow a good used prefrontal lobe to assist her with her insight, foresight, and hindsight.

Post-traumatic stress disorder (PTSD) may come along with a difficult birth (up to 6 percent of the time). It is the second worst combination with BP (trauma and BP). The worst combination is BP and hormones. If it was a traumatic birth, this is liable to wake up the bipolar monster. If this is so, Mom is going to need a stress-free environment as much as possible and treatment for her PTSD (as anyone would who had trauma).

Feedback from the Front

Feedback from mental health-care workers (psychologists, social workers, counselors, nurse practitioners, and M.D.s) over the last eight years indicate that, although hormones and bipolar disorder is usually an exacerbating combination, many women with BP say that they feel great when pregnant. These are women with stable lives who go off their medication slowly for a planned pregnancy, listen to their doctors, research the information available, and plan their pregnancy in advance. Other women who may have unplanned pregnancies, don't know who the father is, or decide to give the baby up for adoption are likely to have more difficulties.

One of the critical periods is after the baby is born. Avoiding the postpartum blues is of significant importance. What may look like postpartum blues may actually be a severe bipolar depression triggered by circadian rhythm changes (changes in sleep pattern).

One way to avoid this is to have someone other than Mom get up with the baby. Maybe Grandma will move in for the first couple of months, or maybe Dad will agree to get up with the baby at night (to avoid his mother-in-law moving in). Mom should be left to sleep through the night. The alternative of making Mom get up with the baby may not be pretty in the long run. Better to set up Mom with help until the baby starts sleeping through the night.

Kristin's Story

Kristin Finn was diagnosed with manic depression as a teenager. Upon deciding to become pregnant, she and her husband had questions, concerns, and fears. Recognizing that there was no go-to guide that helps women with manic depression navigate pre-natal, pregnancy, and postpartum issues, Finn collaborated with geneticists, obstetricians, psychologists, and psychiatrists to write an ultimate support-group-in-a-book and pregnancy resource. She shares her insights and techniques that she developed through two pregnancies, as well as the advice of her esteemed team of experts. For a more in-depth treatment of bipolar pregnancies, see Kristin Finn's book, *Bipolar and Pregnant*.

> **Real People**
>
> "I will always remember the day that Fred and I decided we were going to try to have a baby. It was December 7, 1990: it was a day that continues to shape our lives. I was a medical center representative for a pharmaceutical company at the time. I was traveling for business, staying in a quaint hotel overlooking Lake Michigan. I extended my stay, Fred joined me, and we took this opportunity to focus on our future. The apprehension and uncertainty that we had been feeling was replaced with a surge of peace and joy.
>
> Fred comments as follows: "When Kristin and I started talking about having a baby, I was ecstatic about being a dad. I had always thought I would like to have children, but at the same time I was concerned for Kristin's health. We had no way of knowing how being off lithium would affect her. This was the only Kristin I knew. I felt a mixture of emotions: excitement at the idea of parenthood, but also apprehension about her well-being."
>
> "Although we were unsure of our immediate future, Fred and I were driven to begin this new chapter in our lives. Together we started breaking down this life-changing decision into manageable parts."
>
> —*Bipolar and Pregnant: The first book to tackle one of the leading concerns of women with manic depression and related disorders*, by Kristin Finn. Reprinted by permission from Health Communications, Inc.

The Least You Need to Know

♦ Although bipolar disorder can make pregnancy a bit more challenging, many bipolar women have happy, successful pregnancies and uncomplicated deliveries.

◆ Pregnancy doesn't mean you must go without any meds. There are some BP meds considered safe during pregnancy, so ask your doctor about this.

◆ Moderate exercise during pregnancy can help your moods, alleviate your stress, and help you feel physically better while pregnant.

◆ For the latest information on bipolar pregnancy, check the website information on NAMI, NIMH, and DBSA.

Chapter 19

Red Tape and Legalities

In This Chapter

- ◆ What happens when someone ends up incarcerated?
- ◆ What legal actions can I take to ensure treatment for a loved one when they need it?
- ◆ Important insurance issues that must be addressed
- ◆ The importance of advance directives

In this chapter, we talk about legal issues: disability, insurance, incarceration, and rights. Incarceration sounds horrible, but it can be a blessing in disguise and actually save the life of someone who may be totally out of control. When a person is so manic and out of control that he refuses treatment, it can be a solution to the difficult problem of mania. The jails have now replaced the state mental institutions of yesteryear. In jail, a person with BP is likely to be taken to the medical center and given a cell by himself in a safe environment. He will have access to treatment and medication and will not be able to use drugs. In this chapter, we will discuss the legal issues related to bipolar disorder.

Disability

A person who is disabled because of bipolar disorder is eligible for disability benefits. Disability for bipolar disorder can be difficult because of the intermittent nature of the bipolar monster. It comes and goes for some people. Just because you have bipolar disorder does not mean you are unable to work. Some people can work for months and then have a couple bad weeks. They may have a manic moment, tell off the boss, and get fired. Others can go for years between episodes. Still others have a few days of the month that they cannot work.

Let's look at three true cases of work scenarios.

Example 1

Dave was a good worker. He loved to work. It kept his mind focused. The problem was that he couldn't keep a job long enough to get medical benefits. Many companies do not grant medical benefits until they are sure an employee is going to work out. Dave would inevitably have a manic moment and tell off his boss or get depressed and not come in for a couple days during his probationary period.

Dave was not a difficult case. If he had the right medication, he would be consistent at his work. Can he work? Yes. That is one of the questions on the application for disability benefits. However, the proper answer is, "Yes, he can work, if his bosses would stop firing him long enough for him to get stable."

Example 2

Sharon had an executive job in a large corporation. She had an episode and was hospitalized. After a week, she was stabilized on her medication and went back to work. However, she could not do the work of an executive at that time. An executive needs a working prefrontal lobe to apply insight, foresight, and hindsight.

The convalescence period after a manic episode is usually six to eight weeks. It takes a little longer if a person's medication needs to be switched, as it often does. After a couple months, Sharon's company let her go with a nice severance package. They said, "We are not letting her go because she has bipolar disorder. We are letting her go for nonperformance issues."

Few people understand that it takes a couple months for the prefrontal lobe to come back after an episode. Even then, brain scans show that it may take 100 days for the lobe to completely come back. Luckily, Sharon was able to find another executive job after her lobe came back online, and the company she works for now have themselves an excellent executive.

Example 3

A young woman started work as a telemarketer. When she applied, she told management that she would have some bad days when she would have to stay home. They were short-handed, so they agreed to these terms. The woman ended up being salesperson of the month three months in a row. Some of the other workers became jealous and made comments such as "How can she be salesperson of the month? She's not here half the time!" New management came in and told the woman she would have to come in every day. She did, and ended up telling off a customer and the new management. They fired her—their best salesperson.

Valuing What's Important

In all the preceding scenarios, the people are capable of working and do not need disability benefits. They need understanding. Dave's boss said, "He does twice the work of anyone when he is here, but I just can't let him disrespect me." In all these scenarios, a little bit of understanding, a little help, and a little leniency would have gone a long way. All three of these employers shot themselves in the foot and lost someone valuable.

Of course, some people with bipolar disorder are more advanced in their illness and truly cannot work. Some people also need to be on temporary disability for a year or so while they recuperate from an episode and the aftermath of that episode (which could mean losing their job, insurance, or spouse).

Our system can be very unkind to people with BP. Plenty of people are refused disability benefits, even if they have had hospitalizations and diagnoses from more than one doctor. By the time a person goes through the red tape, refusals, and second requests, months can pass. It is unlikely that someone who is mentally ill will be able to follow through on all this. Without an advocate, the person may end up getting evicted and becoming homeless.

That is not supposed to happen to people with true disabilities. If you are turned down for SSI disability, you are entitled to have an SSI lawyer, free of charge. The lawyer will take a percentage of the back pay. Of course, part of the reason it is so difficult to qualify for disability now is that people have taken advantage of the system and collected disability when they were actually able to work.

Much of this could be avoided if we had a simple way of providing evaluations and medication for bipolar disorder. It would save money as well as adding to the work force and enabling people to maintain some pride about supporting themselves. Most people with bipolar disorder are like everyone else: they want to work. We end up accommodating them in one way or another.

One way people with BP survive is by starting their own businesses. A business of one's own may provide the flexibility a bipolar person needs, and she can always hire someone with a consistent prefrontal lobe.

For more information about bipolar disorder in the workplace, see Chapter 16.

Insurance Issues

One out of seven admissions to the psychiatric ward is for bipolar disorder. More than 19 percent of people with bipolar disorder commit suicide. The suicide rate is actually estimated to be 25 percent if you consider that there are people whose bipolar disorder is undiagnosed when they commit suicide. The suicide rate is highest in the first two years after the onset of bipolar disorder. The main reasons for these staggering figures are …

- Lack of insurance.
- Lack of facilities.
- The law (requiring immediate danger to self or others for an involuntary commitment).
- The wait time in the emergency room.
- Lack of proper treatment.
- Lack of medical doctors treating BP.

A person going through an episode cannot be expected to have the mental capacity to adhere to the rules set up by a managed care company. If she is living by herself and has no relatives to help, she is not likely to know the rules or to fill out the forms correctly. Afterward, there are always the bills that get rejected by the insurer for this or that reason. This makes no sense at all for people who are incapacitated, whether it is from a mental health problem or a physical problem.

Real People

A woman was experiencing extreme agitation from bipolar disorder, including racing, suicidal thoughts. She called the psychiatric ward and asked if they took her insurance. They did. She admitted herself and spent a week there. Then her insurance company told the hospital they wouldn't pay because she hadn't consulted her primary physician before she was admitted. She had never used her insurance before, and, in her state of mind, her insurer expected her to call her primary care physician.

The hospital sent her a bill for over $6,000. This ruined her credit, as she did not have the strength or mental capacity to fight the insurance company's decision or to follow up for some time afterward.

The best solution is to have an advocate for yourself in place. Find a friend or family member whom you can trust to help with your insurance and hospital forms, and who will fight to get you the best care. In the midst of an episode, you will probably not be in any kind of mental state to take this stuff on.

We have heard this over and over again. There is no generosity in insurance companies. Their motivation is to treat as little as possible and to pay for as little of your treatment as is required. Your advocate should know about your medications, the best facilities, and your insurance, and *you* have to research and arrange it beforehand. This is why a treatment plan is necessary for you to attend to before it happens.

Real People

"If I didn't have my parents to help me, I would be dead now." This is a statement from someone who was so incapacitated and agitated after a manic episode that he truly was going to commit suicide. His parents escorted him to the hospital, got him admitted after waiting six hours in the Emergency Room, and filled out the forms for him.

Insurance companies start off with a conflict of interest. You pay them premiums so that they will pay when you are sick. However, their motive is to make a profit (and not pay). There are plenty of horror stories about insurance companies that we won't go into here. There are also a few good stories about ethical insurance companies.

The chances are good that your bipolar disorder will be treated at a dual-diagnosis rehabilitation facility. Over half of the people with BP have a substance-abuse problem, usually from self-medicating BP symptoms. For that reason, it may be a good idea to check the number of days your insurance policy allows for drug and alcohol rehabilitation. Some allow 30 days or fewer. Some insurance companies will allow two visits a year if the substance abuse problem is still apparent. If you have a substance-abuse problem in combination with bipolar disorder, your stay in rehab is likely to be a couple weeks minimum, and if it isn't, it should be.

The National Health Care Anti-Fraud Association (NHCAA) is a private-public partnership whose members include more than 100 private health insurers and public-sector law enforcement and regulatory agencies having jurisdiction over health-care fraud committed against both private payers and public programs. If you feel that your insurance company is obligated to pay your health-care bills and you have tried and failed to get them to pay, you may contact the NHCAA. The NHCAA website is www.nhcaa.org.

Medicare has a good program that allows decent treatment for bipolar disorder, but if you are under 65 and have no insurance, the medical assistance program may be difficult to work with. There may be a long waiting time before seeing a doctor in some states. Your local Mental Health Association should be able to give you some direction. There is also probably a NIMH (National Institute of Mental Health) organization or a chapter of DBSA (Depression and Bipolar Support Alliance) that can help.

At this writing, the whole country is experiencing a shortage of mental health facilities. There is too little profit and too much litigation. The answer, unfortunately, when there is a problem at a facility, is to shut it down. This country also has a shortage of psychiatrists who are able to take patients on short notice.

When more family physicians receive training in bipolar disorder, this will help reduce the number of suicides and enable patients to endure the wait time until they see a psychiatrist. In fact, bipolar disorder can often be treated by a family physician when there are no other medical factors and the patient is in reasonably good health. Again, the problem is the training of our physicians to handle the physiological problems of bipolar disorder.

The United States has one of the poorest health-care systems for bipolar disorder in the developed world. That's why it is important for you to know as much as you can about your disorder and its proper treatment. It is essential that you catch it before it gets so advanced that you lose perspective. Again, a knowledgeable advocate will be a tremendous asset during trying times.

Legal Issues

Our jails have become the mental institutions of the old days. People with mental health issues may end up in jail for a variety of different behaviors. The most predominant charge is "criminal trespassing." For people with BP, the most predominant charges are the use of illegal drugs. BP sufferers may also incur motor vehicle–related violations, such as a DUI (driving under the influence).

A survey of one jail with 1,200 inmates found that about 5 percent of the prison population had been diagnosed with bipolar disorder. It is estimated that another 5 percent were undiagnosed. Most people with BP in jail are not criminals. Without BP, they would not even be in jail.

During mania, a person may be pulled over for speeding. The officer may suspect they are "on" something and search the vehicle. Sometimes it's just the mania, but 57 to 60 percent of people with BP self-medicate with illegal drugs, so the officer is likely to find something. There is also the possibility that the person will be combative and will get charged with resisting arrest or even assaulting an officer. The "assault" can be something as simple as spitting or pointing and touching the officer. If a person hasn't slept, is a little paranoid, and is being interrogated about drugs she hasn't taken, the situation can easily escalate into assault or resisting arrest. The manic person's ego, arrogance, and entitlement may further aggravate the situation.

Another possible reason for incarceration is "terrorist threats," when, for example, a manic person whose brain is connected directly to his tongue says what he feels at the moment to his neighbor. The police show up, and the manic neighbor admits his threats and even makes more in front of the officer. It's off to jail he goes. Similar to this is the example of someone who becomes agitated and loud and makes threats to her spouse. A neighbor or the spouse calls the police and the police may make the person leave the residence and attend anger management or domestic abuse classes. The spouse or neighbor can apply for a Protection from Abuse (PFA) order to keep the bipolar person away from him or her. If the PFA is violated, the person may be arrested and incarcerated.

Then, of course, there are people with BP who are also criminals because they have nurtured a criminal nature. It is likely that about 5 percent of any prison population has been diagnosed with bipolar disorder. A conservative estimate is that at least 4 percent could be released on medication. With regular medication checks, it is unlikely that a person with BP would repeat the acts that got him or her incarcerated in the first place. Most are in jail because they were involved with illegal drugs, and some because they did something while manic that they would never do otherwise.

An old figure for the cost of incarceration is $31,500 a year. It would be a lot less expensive to have the person on parole or probation and check his or her medication weekly. A program to evaluate and put people who had BP on probation safely would save taxpayers between 42 and 46 billion dollars a year if only 4 percent were eligible. That is a conservative figure. If that money were used to research bipolar disorder, we would probably be able to put most people's bipolar disorder in remission within a couple years.

A Good Defense

The best defense for illegal acts committed during an episode has to make sense to the judge, and the judge has to be reassured that it won't happen again. You (or your attorney) may need to educate your judge about bipolar disorder. Even many mental health professionals do not truly understand bipolar disorder, so the likelihood of a judge understanding it without your help is even less. The judge must understand the disorder in forensic terms.

- How is it that you couldn't help doing what you did?
- How can you guarantee that you are not going to do it again?

The judge is usually able to take circumstances into consideration when charging a person for a crime and also when sentencing a person. The judge is commissioned to protect the public. The lawyer would need an argument that assures the judge that the person couldn't help doing what they did (bipolar disorder acted up) and they won't do it again (will take medication) and the public will be safe (medication will be checked to make sure they are taking it).

First, if a person was "insane" (in a legal sense) at the time of the incident, but is not insane now, that is a good beginning for a defense. If a person has bipolar disorder and was never treated for it, that would explain how she did not have control over the situation, whether it was self-medicating with illegal drugs, assault, threats, or even robbery. The defense would have to show that the person did not have a criminal nature and that anything illegal she did was due to the undiagnosed bipolar disorder. The judge may need to be shown that this person's normal state of mind is not criminally inclined.

Second, a bipolar person will have to show how she will ensure that the criminal behavior not happen again. Perhaps she has now been diagnosed and is on medication. The medication must be shown to be working for her. The medication can be checked to ensure that it is being taken. This will ensure the public safety.

The law can take into consideration that you are not to blame for the incident, though you are still responsible. This is actually one of the most profound things you can learn in life. You are not to blame for your bipolar disorder, but you are responsible for it. If you don't take responsibility for it, you may go off your meds and end up in unacceptable situations (jailed, divorced, jobless).

If you take responsibility for your bipolar disorder, you are likely to get better. If you don't, you won't. When someone says, "I can't help it, I'm bipolar," that's hogwash! That person will not get better.

Granted, it may be difficult and challenging to get better. Can you get better? Absolutely! Better and better and better! Is it unfair that you have to take that challenge? Sure it is. Would you rather take responsibility by taking medication and getting help, or would you rather take responsibility by sitting in a smelly jail? Either way, you will be taking responsibility, but in jail you will also be to blame.

You may be able to apply to have your record expunged. Each state offers its own definition of expungement based on different rules and laws. Generally, expungement can be viewed as "removing records from general review" pertaining to a case. The records may not completely disappear and may still be available to law enforcement in the case of a second offense. Most legal systems only allow records to be expunged once.

Rights and Advance Directives

If there is a mental health court in your community, this could be an avenue to getting treatment for your bipolar disorder. A mental health court gets referrals from the other courts with people who law enforcement believes may have a mental illness or substance abuse problem. The mental health court sends the person for an evaluation and then may "sentence" the person to a rehab or a psychiatric ward for treatment. A person cannot be forced to take medication, and anyone who has ego, arrogance, and entitlement may not do so unless forced. Once the laws are broken, this person may have a choice between incarceration and taking medication for bipolar disorder. Most people will choose the latter. At that point, the medication is monitored, and if the person is not taking his medication, he can be incarcerated. The person may resentfully take the medication for a while, and usually (once his prefrontal lobe is functioning again) will agree that it was the best thing for him.

If you are bipolar, you should use mental health services on a regular basis. It is important to remain in treatment even when you are successfully managing your condition. Your visits to the psychiatrist and psychologist may be reduced to a few times a year at some point during your illness, but they should remain regular for monitoring and management.

Since you cannot be sure how your illness may progress over the years, we advise that you establish an advance directive. Advance directives are legal documents you prepare with an attorney that specify how and in what ways you wish to be treated in the event you are unable to make decisions because of illness or incapacity.

A living will is one type of advance directive with which you may be familiar. In a living will, you detail the types of care you want, such as your wish to be an organ donor and your desire to not be resuscitated after your heart stops. Another form of advance directive, called a health-care proxy, designates a loved one who will make decisions about your treatment while you are incapacitated.

The Five Wishes advance directive is one of several combination documents that names a health-care proxy and outlines your wishes for treatment. We advise you to establish a combination document that covers all your bases, including hospitalization as a result of mental illness. Under normal circumstances, people have the right to refuse medical treatments. Doctors require the patient's informed consent, which means they must explain treatment options to the patient. Then the patient decides when and how they want to be treated and agrees to participate in that treatment.

An exception to the informed consent rule is involuntary commitment to a psychiatric facility (see Chapter 14). In such cases you are considered incapable of giving informed consent. In the event you are involuntarily committed, your health-care proxy will help make decisions on your behalf by following your own detailed instructions, which by law must be adhered to. For example, you can dictate that you are not to be subject to electroconvulsive therapy or to a particular medication.

Your attorney should retain a copy of your advance directive and be responsible for providing it to the mental facility in case your health-care proxy is unable to locate her copy. Your regular doctors should each have a copy as well. The mental facility will request your medical records, and your directive should be a part of your record.

In lieu of a legally prepared document, you can obtain advance directive forms from most hospital admission or patient advocate departments. Your local bar association and Mental Health Association office should also be able to provide the forms. Choose who you wish to act as your proxy and make decisions on your behalf, and be sure that person is willing and able to be so designated. Fill out the forms and discuss each point with your proxy. Furnish signed copies to a friend, a family member, and your doctor. Make sure they understand what you want and what you don't want. In some states like Michigan, where there is no living will law, mental health facilities will usually still abide by the choices you set forth in your directive.

Mental Health Power of Attorney

Some states require a mental health power of attorney, which is just like an advanced directive, but specific to mental health care. In some states the psychiatrist or psychologist has to decide whether you should be committed or not and sign the commitment papers. Following are several instances in which a mental health power of attorney is advisable:

- A woman with BP wishes to get pregnant and wants to go off her medication during pregnancy. If she becomes delusional or psychotic, she wants someone she trusts to admit her to a psychiatric facility or to ensure that she gets medication that won't affect the fetus.

- A person who has reached the legal age to refuse treatment may wish to have his parents, psychologist, or psychiatrist monitor him and admit him against his will if he becomes symptomatic. This would help someone who hasn't been able to manage his BP when symptomatic and safeguard him and his loved ones.

- A person on probation or parole may wish to have someone monitor her so that she does not break the terms of her probation or parole. She can then be forced to take medication or admitted to a psychiatric facility against her will when she is symptomatic.

There are other uses for the mental health power of attorney, but these are the main ones.

The Least You Need to Know

- Incarceration can sometimes be a blessing in disguise for a bipolar person who needs immediate help for substance abuse issues or other problems.

- Lack of insurance (or problems with insurance companies) can be a major problem for people with bipolar disorder.

- It's a smart idea to have an advance directive in place, in case you ever need someone else to make health-care decisions on your behalf.

Chapter 20

Damage Control

In This Chapter

- Some universal methods for picking yourself back up
- What to do when you have done irreversible damage
- Plights and recoveries to learn from

There was a commercial on television that said something like, "Otto is a real person, so we hired an artist to help him tell his story." That would be like saying, "Otto has bipolar disorder, so we hired a doctor to help him tell his story."

Who would you rather talk to you about rough bipolar periods—someone who never experienced one or a real person with bipolar disorder? In this chapter, we present firsthand accounts and advice from people who have lived with bipolar disorder.

Robert Anthony

Meet Bob Anthony. He is a mechanic, an author, and a poet. He is bipolar. He has wrestled with the bipolar dragon many times. He is a warrior. In this country we are allowed to know things. You can know about medication without having to be a doctor. (You just can't prescribe medication.)

You are allowed to know about psychology without being a psychologist. (You just can't call yourself a psychologist.)

Bob knows his bipolar dragon, and when it gets riled up or depressed, he knows what to do. He calls in his allies to help him (therapist, doctor, friends, family). He is aware when the bipolar dragon appears over his horizon. He is ready to do battle if he has to. He has tamed the dragon. It was difficult. It took years. It took help. Bob lost a couple of battles, but the dragon is not Bob's master anymore. Bob is the master of the dragon.

Repairing Damage

Our life is a lifelong duel. People who have bipolar cannot imagine what it is like not to have it (until we are properly medicated with sufficient therapy), and people without it cannot imagine what it is like to have it (without an education in bipolar disorder). This creates a communication barrier that I hope to help bridge in this section. We can start this process by trying to see things from the other's perspective.

This section is about repairing damage: damage to ourselves and our relationships from rough times. When it comes to repairing damage done once we have come out of an episode, there are a few things to keep in mind. First, "Prevention is the only cure for making mistakes." Once the damage has been done, we can't undo it. That is to say, if we don't do any damage in the first place, we have saved ourselves and others a lot of trouble.

Having bipolar for 43 years has taught me some basic facts about it. It has been said that anyone can learn from their own mistakes, but a wise person learns from the mistakes of others. It is my deepest hope that what I have learned from my mistakes can help you learn what to do and what not to do. As well, I would hope that it will help you learn what to do after you do make a mistake.

When we misinterpret people's intentions, we act out of a mistaken perception. That is how and when most damage is done. Those who do not have bipolar do not have this misinterpretation problem. Sure, they make mistakes, but we tend to make bigger ones. We can say the rudest, most inappropriate thing without even meaning to be inappropriate.

These kinds of mistakes led me to do the most damage, which I did to myself, believing I was hopeless. I was thinking of myself in my little world, believing that no one would ever understand or love me because of the failures and the mistakes I had made up to my early 20s. I have compiled a list of things to work on to keep these kinds of things from happening. Things that get in the way of establishing, maintaining, and/or repairing relationships are:

◆ False pride: Believing we don't need anyone's help to manage our condition.

◆ Not being honest with ourselves.

◆ Not being honest with others.

◆ Fear of disapproval from others.

◆ Fear of failure at a relationship or of not being able to make things work out, which causes us to do or say things out of assumption, rather than seeing if our fears are even accurate.

◆ Insecurity: We won't speak up or be assertive if we are insecure, and this may lead to frustration and/or anger because our needs go unmet.

◆ Needing everything done our way—never allowing others to be themselves or do things their way.

◆ Assuming we know what will happen before we even try, like giving up before we even start.

I have had bipolar from childhood, and I have made monumental mistakes. I just thought there was something wrong with me that could not be fixed or managed. On one hand, I was right—I needed more than willpower to manage bipolar. But I didn't know I had bipolar until I was 36! Now I see things more clearly. I see things from people's perspective who don't have bipolar, and from those who do. People are all equal based upon what we need, not upon what we have. Some people have things we don't have, and we with bipolar have problems that other people cannot imagine having to live with, but we all have the same needs, though to different degrees. Our emotions are so intense that they can lead us to suicide and unfathomable rage. My point is we need love, we need respect, we need attention, we need support, and we need each other, just as much as anyone without bipolar. So if there is one mistake I want you to learn from that I made, it is not giving yourself enough credit for surviving what we have to deal with.

Most people without bipolar never consider suicide. It happens outside of bipolar, too, but the suicide rate for bipolar is the highest among any illness, or any other cause. Most people can't imagine being driven to the point that suicide looks reasonable. We make mistakes when we are manic or depressed and when we return to normal mode wonder, "What was I thinking?" People without bipolar don't have that problem as much.

Repairing the damage to our self esteem is, I believe, the most important damage to repair. If we don't have self esteem, we cannot progress in repairing damage to relationships, at work, legally, or financially. I only learned how to repair my self esteem by reading Dr. Jay's book, *Nasty People: How to Stop Being Hurt by Them without Becoming One of Them!* That book got me started, and with additional talk therapy and finally medication, the lights came on and I now have a healthy self esteem.

Each person is given his own load to carry. But with bipolar, we are given a boulder to carry that no human being can, could, or ever would be able to carry. We need to understand that we deserve a medal of honor just for surviving. When we have made a mistake in manic mode, the first thing we want to do is beat ourselves up. We tend to really, really want to feel bad about it. Only good people feel bad about what they did wrong. So feeling bad after a rough time is very understandable. But we can't go too far with this because then we turn self-destructive and feed the bad side of us.

Recovering from hard times takes self-discipline to keep from beating ourselves up. We cannot let the fact that we made a mistake keep us from trying to do the right things again. So what if I started smoking again? I can quit again, and the sooner I quit, the easier it is to quit! It is the same with any mistake; the sooner we say, "I apologize," the less we will have to apologize for, the easier it will be to apologize, and the sooner we feel better.

If you believe you just have a more difficult life than other people, but that it doesn't make you a bad person, you are off to a great start. There is a difference between a reason and an excuse. While there are reasons we do things when manic, mixed, or depressed, that doesn't always excuse the things we did. When there are reasons we make mistakes, we can excuse ourselves, but that doesn't mean everyone else will understand or excuse our behavior.

When we punish ourselves, it can be counterproductive. Winners are losers who never stop trying. That is the most important thing to understand about recovering from rough times. We must keep trying to improve our condition. Understand the reason we made a mistake and do what we can to keep it from happening ever again. We do this by telling our doctor when we fouled up, what happened. Were we manic in an extreme way and lost control of our behavior again? Did we become depressed and gave up on our diet again? Did we try to take our own life? Did we become aggressive with someone we love and now feel horrible about it? We need to communicate with our psychiatrist and psychologist the exact nature (or reasons) of our wrongs.

I have been properly medicated now for going on five years. I have felt suicidal, but realized that was not a course of action I wanted to take. There is a huge difference between having a thought or feeling and acting on those thoughts or feelings! I have been manic and spent my money on things I didn't need, but that doesn't mean I just gave up and stopped trying. That is how I have tamed the dragon. We feed the dragon with what we do. If we do good things, he stays tamed; when we start acting on bad thoughts, he grows stronger!

One day I was fortunate enough to run across a great psychiatrist and he worked with me to get my medication straight. I am on one anti-psychotic, two mood stabilizers, two anti-depressants, and one minor tranquilizer! But that is what it takes to keep my dragon tame. I have been in therapy for years, but I will continue and see no end in sight. Why would I change what works?

If you are coming out of a rough time and feel bad, that means you are a good person. Keeping the dragon tamed sometimes requires cracking the whip and doing things you don't want to do, or not doing the things you want to do. Not every person with bipolar has been given the knowledge contained in this book. You are one of the fortunate ones who now have the tools, the knowledge, and the skills it takes to keep that dragon tame. It is up to you to put forth the effort.

Mental Note

More than likely, if you are out of control—losing your temper, driving recklessly, taking exceptional risks—your medication is not adequate. I still feel like screwing up, I just don't do it. I still feel suicidal at times, I just don't act on it! If you do not have this kind of control, you are either insufficiently medicated or you are not trying the right way.

Be honest with your doctor about *all* of your problems. If you are doing something that is beyond your control, it means you need medication. It is a biological problem, not a personality problem. People don't look down on people with cancer, diabetes, or paraplegia. Some people may have looked down on you, but there is no difference between a diabetic and a person with bipolar other than the kind of chemicals we need to stabilize us. The only thing difference is they need chemicals (insulin) for their body, and we need chemicals (various medications) for our brain.

The Importance of a Support Network

Like I said earlier, we can't cross a bridge that has been burned, but we can build a new bridge. We do this by first establishing a strong personal support network. It cannot be over-stressed that people with bipolar, including me, need to have close friendships with many people.

People with bipolar need a support network for the following reasons:

◆ We need someone to ask if our judgment has been or is distorted.

◆ We need someone to point out to us when we are in an episode so we know to take appropriate action. Even if we don't see or perceive that we are, they can tell better than we can when we are going into an episode.

◆ We need someone to manage our money in most cases.

◆ We need someone to be accountable to.

◆ We do better not living alone. I don't suggest living alone if it is not necessary. And if we do live alone we need a good support network of people that we can talk to daily that know us well and can be sounding boards for our plans, ideas, and thoughts.

Patricia C. Friel

This section is written by Patricia C. Friel, M.S., Professional Clinical Counselor, and Licensed Independent Chemical Dependency Counselor. Her M.S. is in mental health counseling and is from Wright State University in Dayton, Ohio. She is the author of *Aspects of Personal Faith: Personality and Religion in Western and Eastern Traditions.*

Repairing Relationships: One Woman's Story

People with bipolar disorder can have healthy relationships—once the person who is bipolar is stabilized. At least, that has been true for me. It also takes active, intentional family involvement to learn about the disease and to learn how to communicate with the person who has the disease. However, many times relationships are so irrevocably damaged while the disease is in its active phase that the relationships dissolve into resentment, anger, ostracization, and divorce if appropriate intervention does not take place in time. I speak from personal experience.

Hi! My name is Pat and I have bipolar disorder. I had my first full cycle at age 18, but was not diagnosed until my late twenties. I was married at 21; my husband was 25. Two more different personalities who came together would be hard to find. I was happy-go-lucky, laughed at everything (both appropriate and inappropriate), could be considerate or inconsiderate, and could be obnoxious or deeply caring. I could be clingy or extremely strong-willed and independent. These traits only worsened with time. My husband was a quiet, easygoing man and in control of himself at all times. I enjoyed his calmness and he liked my spontaneity. That was then. After a year or two of marriage, the qualities that brought us together started the inexorable slide into slowly driving us apart.

We have been married 37 years. Part of it has been eternal bliss and part hell on earth, and the rest, of course, everything in between. Because I was a rapid cycling bipolar, neither my husband nor I would know the mood I would be in on any given day when he came home from work. Then, there would be times I wouldn't even be there. He would be lucky if I had left a note to let him know I'd taken off on a trip across the United States or had once again been admitted to the hospital.

Over the years, as my anger and paranoia built, I learned to live a very secret life. I also tried to keep my disease a secret from other people because I felt so much shame and guilt. One of the biggest problems, as I saw it at the time, was that my husband did not seem interested in the disease or want to discuss it. I felt I was carrying the load by myself. I felt that his attitude was, if you don't talk about it, it will go away. I became more secretive and withdrawn from him. The gaps in our communication became more strained. I felt I was to blame for my disease and the stigma it carried. I prayed to be healed so that I would not have to take medications that had side effects I did not like or that simply did not work. Other people that I trusted with my "secret" prayed. Time and time again, I went off medication because as I cycled into feeling hypomanic, I felt I had been healed—only to crash again after a few weeks or go into a full-blown manic state. So much for prayer and self-control! And during most of that time I was in total denial that I was bipolar.

As time went on, the uncertainty of the disease wore out both of us and took an enormous toll on our marriage. At times, I would be very paranoid and angry with him. Of course, I always had valid reasons in my mind to support my thoughts, feelings, and subsequent behaviors. At other times, I would put him on a pedestal. I could rarely see beyond a given moment to put our relationship into perspective. Communication at all levels eroded. In between my bipolar swings, our relationship would struggle to return to "normal," but the normal phases became farther and farther apart. Finally, communication became nil at times.

After receiving my Master's degree in my late 40s, I left him—sort of! I moved an hour and a half away to a new job, but would come home every weekend to do laundry and clean house. There was little communication between us at that time beside "How was your week?" "Fine, how was yours?" "Fine." Then I would return to my new home. The next weekend, I would be back for the same routine, still paranoid, angry, resentful, and furious at him.

This lasted about two years. Our relationship stayed static for about three years. I was quite self-supporting and self-sufficient with few major mood swings. However, the toll of a high-stress job teamed with perfectionist tendencies soon ate away at my semi-stable condition. I slowly sank into a very deep depression. I did not eat or sleep. I could not function enough to go to work, so I took a leave of absence. I moved back in with my husband and continued to deteriorate, and once again ended up in the hospital. The doctors ordered a series of electroconvulsive treatments, which ended up lasting for two years. Whether due to ECTs, medication changes, or menopause, I slowly recovered from the depression and experienced fewer violent and abrupt mood swings.

To make a long story short, my healing and the healing of our marriage didn't take place until I took the first step of a 12-step program. I admitted I was powerless over my disease and my life had become unmanageable. (A friend who was in recovery suggested I try the program.) It was so freeing to finally recognize that I had a disease and that I was not responsible for my mood changes. The denial was gone. I could finally deal with my bipolar disorder. My feelings of shame, guilt, and embarrassment have slowly receded. I have learned to look my disease square in the face. I learned to be honest with myself about my feelings. I could finally learn to be honest with my husband about our relationship. That meant we had to go back decades to begin to repair all the real and imagined hurts of our marriage.

Because of my work in the mental health and substance abuse fields, I learned about good communication skills. We began to use "I" statements instead blaming "you" statements when discussing our past relationship difficulties. We stopped blaming each other and began to take personal responsibility for our past feelings and behaviors. The last three or four years have been a time of healing. We started setting time aside during my lengthening stable times to discuss past misunderstandings and hurts. We gave each other the freedom to be totally honest. No topic was off-limits.

Those discussions opened the door for me to realize he loved me and cared about me, and that I loved him and cared about him, also. This honesty has led to us trusting each other as we never had in the past. One of the hardest areas of trust, for me, was giving him permission to help monitor my mood swings. I not only gave him permission to help monitor me, but promised to listen to him when he suggested I needed to call the doctor. I recognized that I do not think clearly when I am manic or severely depressed. I had to learn to trust him to help monitor me. It is difficult to listen because I like the rush being slightly manic gives me. Because I am now trusting his input, he has learned to trust me: to trust that I will not engage in self-defeating behaviors and to know I will listen and follow through with his suggestions—not react with anger.

The hardest thing to live up to is listening to him and following his advice. I still get very headstrong and rebellious when I'm manic and really don't want to listen to anyone's advice. Secrecy and dishonesty can no longer be a part of our relationship. Recriminations are in the past once we resolved the old issues. It has helped tremendously for him to become an active, intentional participant in gaining knowledge about the disease, and it has made me feel it is a demonstration of his love for me. That is healing for our relationship.

I once read that there are four stages of marriage: romance, disillusionment, the power struggle to change your partner back to who he or she was when you first met, and a couple—two separate entities, but one. We are now a couple. Healing is still taking place, but trust and communication are now paramount in our relationship.

I give God all the thanks and glory for allowing us to work through this disease and for both of us to come to terms with it. There are still times when I could find it easy to slip back into the old habits of not communicating and not trusting, but as time goes on and I practice the new communication patterns I have learned, it becomes easier for old thoughts, feelings, and behaviors to pass into yesterday.

Yes, repairing relationships can be accomplished. Hang in there and God bless!

Thoughts from Jay Carter

It seems that the bipolar monster hides, at first. Even when we think we see the monster, we don't want to believe it: "I am not 'mentally ill.'" And you may not be mentally ill, but you may have bipolar disorder. The monster shows more and more of himself, until we finally accept that he is there. We can do battle with him once he comes out of hiding. Then you have to ask yourself if you are going to be a warrior or a wimp. Warriors get bruises. They get hurt. But wimps do, too. It depends on whether you want to rise from the ashes or hide in the ashes.

Sometimes it takes a long time to finally get to the point where you are accustomed to battling the monster. You will get better and better at it as time goes on. We have good "spotters" now. The monster gets identified sooner. We have better "potions" now, and better ones coming. I have hopes for a potion that makes the bipolar monster disappear or that at least locks him up. But even then, there will be those who want to tease him and get him riled up for the excitement of it. I want to see bipolar disorder cured or totally managed before my lifetime is over. I think we are within 10 years of doing that if we direct the resources to it.

There are warriors, and then there are warriors' warriors. A few good warriors' warriors are in this book. Let's tame the bipolar monster before the next 10 years pass. Don't give up. Return his "gifts," put out his flame, and kick his butt.

The Least You Need to Know

- You are not alone.

- Help is there. Seek it and you will find it.

- A moment that feels like forever will pass.

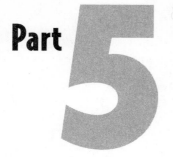

Part 5

For Families

This part of the book is dedicated to the friends and relatives of people with bipolar disorder. We'll tell you how to best help your loved one and what you can do to make things easier for him or her.

Chapter 21

Getting Help for Your Bipolar Family Member

In This Chapter

- ◆ Taking responsibility
- ◆ Communicating effectively
- ◆ Advocating for your BP loved one

If you have a family member with bipolar disorder, you probably want to help him or her, but you may not know how. This chapter will tell you how you can be a good "helper" for your bipolar loved one.

Author Jay watched his beloved child experience mania manifesting as agitation. He saw the frightened look in her eyes, and felt the powerlessness the mania evoked. Then also, his child experienced euphoric mania, including ego, arrogance, and entitlement she had never before shown. The proper thing to do during any episode is to be loving and caring and keep the communication going. Maintain the connection you have with your loved one. When the words and the behavior don't make sense, the only thing you can do is stay connected.

Getting Started

Getting help for a loved one who has bipolar disorder may be one of the most difficult things you have to do. It is painful to watch your family member go through a bipolar episode. If your loved one is experiencing his or her first episode, you may have no idea where to start or who to go to, and you may have no understanding of the disorder. If you have been through an episode with your loved one before, you have learned some things to expect, but you can still improve your knowledge base.

Treatment for BP includes an expected confidentiality between doctor and patient. In order for the doctor to talk to you, the patient has to sign a release of information form. It is very helpful if you can:

- ◆ Get your family member to sign off on the confidentiality agreement, with regard to:

  a. Discussing his medications with the doctor.

  b. Allowing you to attend some of his appointments.

  c. Enabling you to talk to facilities representatives about his treatment.

  d. Including the rest of the family in decisions about finances, facilities, treatment, and type of therapy.

- ◆ Assure the patient that you will not be privy to any of the very private details of therapy. Put this in writing in the confidentiality release. Do this at the outset of treatment, or if you can't, keep trying.

- ◆ Ask the doctor if you can give your input, with the understanding that the doctor may not be able to give you any information in return.

It has been shown that the best therapeutic outcomes happen when the family and significant others are involved in treatment. Any private conversations the patient has with the doctor should be held in confidence; however, with bipolar disorder, the perspectives of those who know the patient can be enlightening to the doctor.

The Health Insurance Portability and Accountability Act (HIPAA) was enacted by the U.S. Congress in 1996. HIPAA protects health insurance coverage for workers and their families when they change or lose their jobs. It also requires the establishment of national standards for electronic health care and addresses the security and privacy of health data. The patient will be asked to sign a document confirming that he has seen the privacy provisions, usually before any consultation is given. Next, if it is agreed that you will participate in the treatment, the patient signs a release of information, specifically denoting the type of information that will be released to you by the doctor so you can track the treatment.

The Proper Approach

Our mental health system is set up to protect the confidentiality of the patient. This is almost always a good thing, except when the patient needs more help than the doctor can provide. It can be frustrating to a loved one who *knows* this patient. With bipolar disorder, the most successful treatment outcomes seem to be when the loved ones are involved. Privileged information, such as sexual history or illegal drugs used, may be shameful to the patient and is only useful in therapy. Reassure the patient that you will not be told anything that is private between the patient and doctor. In most states, parents have a right to know any information about their children up to a certain age (this varies by state).

Still, it is not a good idea to press the doctor or therapist for this privileged information that should remain confidential between patient and doctor. The client may shut down and refuse to reveal certain things to the doctor, which would impede therapy. The therapist may suggest that the patient divulge this information to her parents, but it should be the patient's choice.

The preceding works very nicely. However, sometimes our mental health rules can impede the resolution of a serious matter when there is an exception and lives are at stake.

Emergency Care During Pregnancy

A young bipolar woman decided she wanted to have a baby. She discussed it with her husband and doctor and went off her medication slowly. The doctor suggested taking medication during pregnancy, but the young woman wouldn't hear of it. She didn't want her child exposed to any kind of drugs. Her husband agreed.

Shortly after becoming pregnant, the young woman started having trouble sleeping. She was working in a stressful job, and sometimes she wouldn't sleep all night. Her husband suggested that she see her doctor for medication, but she refused. It wasn't long before she had a full-blown manic episode and took the credit cards to fly out to California.

In California, she met a drug dealer, decided he was her "soul mate," and moved in with him. She began using cocaine, ecstasy, and alcohol. She called her mother to tell her she had met her soul mate and her mother became very upset and called several psychiatrists in the area. They all told her the same thing: "If she is not a danger to herself or others, we cannot admit her against her will. The fetus is not a legal person under the law, so she can't be admitted for being a danger to her baby." This went on for a few days.

Finally, the mother called a psychiatrist with a soft heart and told him that her daughter had threatened to kill her. The doctor admitted the daughter involuntarily and put her on haloperidol, which is rated as "insignificant" for causing birth defects. After a couple days, the young woman became lucid and her mother flew out to bring her home.

The young woman didn't remember much about her manic experience. She knew her mother had done the right thing by lying to the doctor, saving her life and the life of the baby. In her right mind, she never would have taken drugs. She worked things out with her husband and they had a healthy baby.

However, after that, the young woman stayed away from her mother as much as possible. They had been close, and in therapy, when she was asked why she avoided her mother, she broke into tears and said, "Because she betrayed me."

Trying to Fit into the System

Am I trying to get at something here? Yes. On its face, it seems ridiculous for the young woman to have this attitude toward her mother. The young woman was ashamed of herself, but she still had a hard time being in her mother's presence. She couldn't help it.

When a person becomes that manic, she may be overwhelmed. Being overwhelmed is exactly what causes post-traumatic stress disorder. When overwhelmed, the body goes into survival mode. The young woman suppressed the betrayal and it became an unexpressed emotion. Feelings will stay with you until you express them. With eye movement desensitization and reprocessing (EMDR) therapy, she was finally able to release the trauma. Weird, huh? Complicated reactions like these are yet another reason why people with BP are not understood.

The greatest rules can impede the purpose they were designed to assist. People with bipolar disorder can be misunderstood when there is actually a valid reason for their reaction. People with bipolar disorder are square pegs who have trouble fitting in the round holes of our mental health system.

Communication Is Key

Your loved one's doctors or therapists may not be able to talk to you about her case, but you can certainly talk to them. What you say and how you say it can be very important. The doctors are looking for certain symptoms, and sometimes it is difficult for them to see those symptoms if your loved one gives them a different impression. Bipolar people often manage to appear "just fine" in front of the doctor.

How does the doctor know that she hasn't slept for days, and in general doesn't sleep very much at all? You tell the doctor. How does the doctor know that he talks so rapidly that you sometimes can't make out what he's saying? You, again. How does the doctor know your family member becomes very agitated and has bouts of rage? Right, you.

The problem is that when a person is having bipolar symptoms, his perspective is skewed (if he is able to have perspective at all). The patient may believe he is getting enough sleep and say he feels rested. He may agree that he could control his anger better, but not that he intimidates people. He may admit he gets a little moody sometimes. He isn't necessarily lying. He may really perceive his actions that way; furthermore, it's only human to minimize one's extreme behavior to save face.

Bipolar "Anger"

People with BP get angry just like anyone else. When a person is angry, sometimes it is best to just let her rant for a while, until she gets her feelings out. Then you can talk. However, if it's not really anger, but rather bipolar rage, letting her rant is not a good idea. Adrenaline and mania are not a good combination. They contribute to an endless loop effect that gets worse and worse the longer it goes on.

Where there is mania, there are mood swings. You may be able to use this to your advantage. This author's mother had bipolar disorder and I learned to switch her moods with humor. I would exaggerate something, dramatize something, or distract her attention. I might point out the window and say, "Look! Mrs. Scott's butt got really big!" Once my mother looked, she was switched. She might laugh or say, "Now, don't make fun of other people."

A person can develop a great sense of humor this way. For as intense as it may seem at the moment, a bipolar rage can easily switch to another emotion. I used this technique not only with my mother, but also at a jail I was at (as a staff member, of course) for two and a half years.

There is also a "transfer technique" that seems to work on bipolar irritable rage. This technique won't work if there is an obsession about the object of anger that goes along with the mania. However, you may be able to distract the person within the context of the obsession. My mother was obsessed with our getting good grades in school, especially when she was manic. If I showed up with a bad report card on a manic day, she would go on and on and on in a lecture that never ended.

I remember once distracting her by saying, "Did you know that Jeff [my brother] got a D in geometry?" She said, "What?!" and I knew I had transferred her obsession to him. That's pretty low, but I was a teenager. I then was able to leave, knowing she would lie in wait for my brother.

My technique has improved over the years. I might now try to transfer a bipolar person's obsession into the political arena. There is such a variety of misbehavior among political figures that you are sure to find one who will match the object of a person's obsessions.

Bipolar Depression

Depression is a difficult thing to talk about. People with BP can be so intelligent and articulate that they may sound very convincing as they explain why they should just jump off the Golden Gate Bridge and get it over with. "My life has been horrible," a bipolar loved one might tell you. "It's horrible now, and it will never change."

This is where you get to be your loved one's prefrontal lobe for a while, reminding him of the bigger picture he may be incapable of seeing for the moment. The thing to avoid is getting personally caught up in the negativity. Remind him that he is unable, at the moment, to see the bigger picture. Remind him of the blessings he has in life. Name these things. Reassure him that he has people who love him. He may get a glimpse of the bigger picture and that may provide a little bit of hope to get through the rough time.

A person who is depressed after an episode may tell you that he can't think straight. Assure him that, though his prefrontal lobe is off-line temporarily, it will come back online in six to eight weeks. Remind him that he cannot see the purpose in life because there is no prefrontal lobe to see it with. When it comes back (and it will), he will be able to see it again. Tell him that though it seems this state will last forever, it won't.

Keep in mind that the person is not seeing the bigger picture. Have patience for things he says or does that ordinarily would be perceived as selfish, rude, or petty. You may have to try to imagine what it's like to be in your loved one's state of mind. Try to imagine life without a prefrontal lobe. That part of you that sees what you are thinking isn't operating, so you might just say whatever you are thinking. That part of you that sees what you are feeling and decides whether to show the emotion isn't there, so your emotions just comes out. If a person who has been there for you does something that annoys you, you go off on him because you are incapable of seeing the bigger picture of all that he has done for you.

Real People

A father was very close to his daughter. He knew her. One day she became agitated and began exhibiting the ego, arrogance, and entitlement of bipolar disorder. A doctor diagnosed her with a personality disorder, but the father knew that wasn't correct.

The medication the doctor put her on, however, was also a good medication for bipolar disorder. After a while, the "personality disorder" disappeared. In this case, the misdiagnosis didn't matter, as long as the medication did the job. The father knew the medications well enough to keep his mouth shut and his daughter got treated for her bipolar disorder.

The daughter's explanation of her experience (losing the lobe) was very enlightening. She said, "It's like I am the captain on the ship of my life and I am steering the ship where I want it to go. Then the rudder breaks and I can't steer the ship anymore, but the engines are still running fast."

What If My Loved One Doesn't Want Help?

If your loved one needs help, but her judgment is so poor that she doesn't realize how deteriorated she is, you may have to get help in having her hospitalized against their will. It is easiest to do this with an underage child. It is much more difficult to do this with someone who is of legal age. Someone of legal age must be an immediate danger to herself or others before she can be involuntarily hospitalized.

Taking Control

There is only so much you can do, even if you know that a loved one needs help badly, and even if you know he or she will deteriorate further without it. This is one of the problems with our health-care system. It doesn't work well for people with bipolar disorder. That's why the suicide rate is so high for people with bipolar disorder. That's why people with bipolar disorder are left to ruin their lives, gambling away their savings, destroying their marriages, and so on. You may know that a person is going to crash from the mania into a deep, dark depression, but there may be little you can do.

One mother antagonized her manic legal-age son to get him help. She finally said, "I bet you would like to shoot me, wouldn't you?"

He said, "You bet I would!"

She told the police that her son had threatened to shoot her and they admitted him for homicidal threats.

A 14-year-old in the middle of a manic episode would sneak out at night and meet boys for sex. She was doing all kinds of drugs. She was uncontrollable and told her mother, "Just leave me alone and let me live my life the way I want to." She was at high risk for pregnancy, diseases, overdose, and death.

Her mother had her committed to a special school for girls 60 miles away from home. She could not leave the grounds. She did not have access to her usual "friends." She was put on medication for bipolar disorder. She spent a year at the school, feeling resentful and abandoned by her mother.

Eight years later, she is best friends with her mom. She takes her medication consistently. She has a good relationship with a nice man.

Most of the time, if you can get a child through adolescence alive, without the baggage of pregnancy or disease, a better day will come. This young girl had a severe case of mania with hypersexuality. She needed to be in a safe place, and her mother could not provide that for her because of the intensity of her mania. Unbeknownst to her mother, she had also been sexually molested at an early age, which exacerbated her bipolar disorder.

Doing the best thing for your child doesn't mean that your child will like you for it. It can be extremely difficult. The child knows what buttons to push to make you feel like a monster. In the case of this young girl, the years after she left the school were still rocky, but she was somewhat more contained. She has perspective now and realizes that her mother probably saved her life. With therapy and the right medication, she is able to live her life in a more stable way and has a future.

Incarceration

This may sound ludicrous, but sometimes incarceration is a life-saving event. It is sometimes the only way to get help for someone who is deteriorating rapidly. Given that almost 20 percent of people with BP end up committing suicide, the big-picture question you may have to answer is, "Would I prefer to see my loved one in jail or dead?"

Fifty-seven to 60 percent of people with BP abuse substances. This can be advantageous if the only way to save someone's life is to have her incarcerated. Maybe she will only stay one night in a holding area. Maybe she will end up in jail. Either alternative may help.

If your loved one is going before a judge, find out which judge and write a one-page letter. Yes, one page. Call the judge's office, get the fax number, and fax in your letter requesting that the judge order a psychiatric evaluation. The judge may make this a condition of probation and may add to the terms of the probation that the psychiatrist's recommendations have to be followed.

If your loved one ends up in jail, write a one-page letter to the jail's medical department, listing the symptoms (from the DSM-IV) that your loved one exhibits, and ask that your loved one be assessed for mental health problems. Send it certified mail with a return receipt to make sure the medical department sees it. Mail can get backed up in the medical department of a jail.

Your Rights and Responsibilities

It's important for you to be educated and informed about your rights and responsibilities with regard to bipolar children or family members.

Rights of Parents Regarding Children

The Supreme Court has ruled that parents have a fundamental right to control the upbringing and education of their children and that laws or governmental actions that unreasonably infringe upon the rights of parents to raise and educate their children according to their own values are constitutionally suspect.

In most states, parents do not have a right to their child's mental health information unless the child is incapacitated by mental retardation or extremely young. The decision to release this information is usually up to the attending therapist, doctor, or psychiatrist, and must be in the interest of the child.

Responsibilities of Parents Regarding Children

In some states it is considered a crime when parents or guardians do not "exercise reasonable care, supervision, protection, and control" over their children. A parent can be fined for a child being truant, damaging property, or hurting another, for example, in certain states.

The keyword is "reasonable" control over children. There is likely to be more legislation that makes parents responsible for the actions of their children. These laws can put a parent in a double bind. For example, you can drive your child to school and make sure that the child goes inside, but you can't control it if your child then runs out the back door. If your child has BP along with a social phobia, school can be difficult.

The U.S. Department of Health and Human Services provides a National Mental Health Information Center under the Substance Abuse and Mental Health Services Administration (SAMHSA) that provides free information about child and adolescent mental health. Each state has its own treatment programs for children and adolescents. SAMHSA has a toll-free number and its website is www.samhsa.gov. Information can also be obtained from the National Alliance on Mental Illness (NAMI) website at www.nami.org.

Other Family Members

In the case of an elderly loved one with bipolar disorder, legal documents appointing you as his or her temporary guardian should be drawn up. In lieu of this, the patient should sign a "release of information" form, so you can monitor, contribute, and advocate for him or her.

In this country, we perceive ourselves first as individuals. In other countries, people perceive themselves first as family. Bipolar disorder is genetic. If you are in the family and you didn't get BP, you are lucky. And there aren't too many families where one person's BP doesn't affect the rest of the family. It is a family problem. When families (rather than individuals) are treated for bipolar disorder, the outcomes are much more successful.

Caring for the Caregiver

The third step in a 12-step program is "surrender." One definition of *surrender* is "to yield to the power of another." It doesn't mean you just wimp out. It means that …

1. You do everything you can do.

2. You do what is appropriate.

3. Then you leave it up to a higher power.

It doesn't mean that you quit. If something comes up that you can do and if it's appropriate to do it, then you do it. Once you have realized that you do not have ultimate power over the situation, you can have some peace about it.

Your alternative is to worry. To worry is to assume a responsibility that is not necessarily ours to assume. Worry often carries with it the notion that you are the only one who can do anything about a situation, along with a feeling of powerlessness. Don't worry! It accomplishes nothing and stresses you out so your energy is sapped when there *is* something you can do.

Try to get this concept over to your loved one when they are lucid. Be responsible to yourself and your own well-being. Responsibility is a choice. Some people do not choose to be responsible for their bipolar disorder. Okay, so it's unfair. An "I am not going to deal with this" attitude will make a person end up dealing with it, dealing with it, and dealing with it. They can deal with their bipolar disorder once, or they can deal with it again and again; one way or another, they will be dealing with it. Things usually go more smoothly if they take responsibility for them.

Caregiving can be stressful. Sustained, elevated levels of the stress hormone cortisol can put caregivers at risk of physical health problems. When you are under the stress of providing care and advocacy for your loved one, make sure you have enough help and take breaks whenever you can. Develop a "healthy selfishness." If you don't take care of yourself, you may not be able to help as effectively.

The Least You Need to Know

♦ Taking responsibility for things is a choice and gives you more power to affect them than just being a bystander.

♦ Maybe you didn't go to medical school, but you are allowed to know things about medication and treatment.

◆ You may have to make some very difficult choices to save the life of your loved one, and you may not be liked for what you do. Inform yourself as best you can, and do what you feel is right.

◆ Get involved in the treatment of your loved one. Never mind if you are a pain. Be respectful but assertive—you don't have to be "nice."

Chapter 22

Living With a Partner Who's Living With Bipolar Disorder

In This Chapter

- ◆ What you feel is totally normal!
- ◆ Deciding what is you and what is bipolar disorder
- ◆ Avoiding caretaking
- ◆ Protecting yourself financially
- ◆ Creating a loving and stable relationship

This chapter was written by Julie A. Fast, the author of *Loving Someone with Bipolar Disorder: Understanding and Helping Your Partner*. Julie's partner, Ivan, was diagnosed with Bipolar I in 1994. Julie was diagnosed with Bipolar II in 1995. Many years later, they both manage their illnesses daily and are happy to report they have successful relationships in all areas of life.

The First Things You Need to Know

Partners of people with bipolar disorder try to help, want to leave, get upset, fear for their futures, worry about having children, and often love someone so much that it just breaks their heart to see them suffer. As a partner of someone with bipolar disorder, you may know and accept that bipolar disorder is an illness, but when you're on the receiving end of the confusing behavior, you may feel your partner should just be able to control what he or she says and does. Society tells us that an affair is a choice, spending the 401(k) is just stupid, and that staying in bed all day is laziness! But this just isn't reality when a person has bipolar disorder. These are all just normal symptoms of the illness.

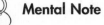

Mental Note

People with bipolar disorder want to get better. They would get well if they could. They have absolutely no desire to have these mood swings, and they need your help.

Before this all makes you feel hopeless and overwhelmed, rest assured that relationships can definitely be loving and committed even when one person has bipolar disorder. Having a successful treatment plan often takes care of so many relationship "problems." Many treatment suggestions are quick and the results are immediate. Others may take much longer and may be lifelong, such as recognizing, modifying, and avoiding triggers, but once the skills are understood, they can be used forever to maintain as stable a relationship as possible.

When Your Partner Has Bipolar Disorder

Love and sex can create wonderful emotions and a bond that is only felt in a romantic relationship. Unfortunately, bipolar disorder could care less about your desires and dreams for a relationship. If untreated, it's a relentless, lifelong illness that has to be controlled in order for you and your partner to create and maintain a stable relationship. This means examining the role bipolar disorder currently plays in your relationship and then finding a way to communicate and grow as a couple, despite the illness that has to be the number-one priority of your relationship.

The facts are that with the correct management tools, this illness can be minimized and controlled, but the mood swings don't simply go away. They are always lurking! You may think, "Wait a minute here! I didn't sign up for this!" No, you didn't, but if you care about your partner and want to keep the relationship strong, changes have to be made. The good news is that many couples say that working on the illness together actually improves their communication skills to the point that they are able to notice and correct behaviors more easily than those couples who don't have the challenge of bipolar disorder. Your goal is for people to say, "His partner may have bipolar disorder, but I've never seen a couple who are more open and loving in their communication."

What You May Experience

As you've learned throughout this book, bipolar disorder is an illness that makes it difficult for your partner to regulate emotions. In fact, you have probably experienced many of the moods your partner experiences. The difference is that your moods are a normal response to a situation. The problem with bipolar disorder is that your partner's moods may be completely unrelated or even abnormal reactions to events. Here are some examples of the differences between your moods and those of your partner.

Example 1

Imagine yourself on the road after a bad day at work. There's a lot of traffic, and then some jerk cuts you off. You may raise your voice, flip the bird, yell out the window, and bang on your steering wheel. But you just keep driving anyway and make it home safely. Though this may be a bit childish, your reaction is pretty common and is a response to an actual event.

Now, imagine all of those feelings and behaviors *without the traffic jam*. Imagine being upset by a stranger walking innocently down the street and then imagine having the thought, "I'm going to beat the #$%$# out of this guy." There isn't even one part of you that says, "If you do this, you may ruin your life. What will happen to your wife? What about your children if you go to jail?" That reasoning is 100 percent gone when your partner is in a violent mood swing. What would it feel like if the emotions and behaviors just showed up with no cause? How would *you* control them in the moment?

Example 2

Remember what it's like when someone breaks up with you—the crying, pain, sadness, despair, worry, and lack of hope that you will ever find someone to love you again. Maybe you stayed in bed for days or missed work. Maybe you cry so hard and so often that you have a fleeting idea that you can't go on this way. Now, imagine having all of those feelings without the breakup! This is what depression feels like. It can be so sudden and so awfully real and intense. And there are often no events that cause the depression. It just shows up and makes your partner miserable—much like the way a person gets pneumonia. Depression really makes you feel like you've been sucker punched in the stomach by life.

Example 3

And finally, can you recall doing something that just made you feel on top of the world? Maybe a concert with your favorite band or a major award? Did you think rationally at that moment? Did you do things such as screaming in joy and trying to rush the stage? Did you feel so much pride that you could literally feel your ego grow? Or how about the elation you felt after the birth of a child that was so great you couldn't stop smiling and maybe even crying in joy? Now, take away the event of the concert or the birth of your child, but keep the elation. That is euphoric mania. It is amazing when it starts and scary and horrific when it gets out of control, and yet for many people, it can just start spontaneously.

These are just three examples from the hundreds of symptoms your partner may experience. The more you can understand bipolar disorder and put yourself in the place of your partner, the more sympathetic you can be to what he or she goes through. And your partner goes through a lot. These unexpected and often out-of-control emotions wear a person out. It's like being flung from a roller coaster when someone has a serious manic episode and finally comes home and has to come down. The main problem is that the feelings *you* experience when your partner goes through this are often ignored. Getting your partner stable is all that matters. And yet, you are the one who takes care of him or her when he or she is sick. His or her behavior affects you in so many ways it's often hard to even remember what your relationship was like when it started. This means that while your partner is getting stable, you have to find a way to keep yourself stable at the same time.

What About You?

According to Dr. John Preston, my coauthor on *Take Charge of Bipolar Disorder* and the author of *The Complete Idiot's Guide to Managing Your Moods*, the following are the main areas where you may have trouble in your relationship.

◆ Your partner is moody, irritable, depressed, and often compulsive. Because of this, there is a loss of a dream of the long-term relationship you anticipated based on what you saw in your partner before your partner became ill.

◆ Your partner experiences ups and downs in sexual behavior (desire) due to the illness or medication side effects. Perhaps your partner doesn't want to be touched. Or he or she is reckless sexually because of mania. You may also lack sexual attraction to your partner because he or she has gained weight due to medication side effects.

Real People

When my partner, Ivan, started to get manic, the manic behavior came in spurts. He beat up a stranger on a train track in Japan, where we were living at the time. He called me from the police station. I was so shocked! He is the most gentle person I've ever known. It just didn't make sense. Then he slept with one of his students. He was mortified and had no idea what happened. He didn't tell me because he was so ashamed of himself.

He went back to his normal self after this. We moved to the States a few months later and he took a job at Microsoft. Things started to fall apart immediately. The move was too big of a trigger and the mania, which was obviously agitated mania, started to take over even more. He had trouble at work and just couldn't get his bus schedule straight. He was so nervous and unhappy. I assumed it was just culture shock, as he's from France.

The night before he went into the hospital, he couldn't remember how to write a check and had trouble counting money. When I woke up the next morning, he was sitting at our kitchen table writing a software program that he said was going to "revolutionize Microsoft and the world!" He's an incredibly intelligent man, so I just assumed he meant what he said. He looked funny, though. His eyes were wild and he looked pretty tired. I, of course, had no idea the grandiose manic thoughts were starting.

Believe it or not, it was his birthday and we had planned a big party. That morning he just wouldn't stop talking. He told me how to park the car even though he couldn't drive! He told my brother he could fix his relationship and he told us that he had the answers to all communication problems. We all just said, "What is up with Ivan? This is not like him." He started to get incoherent a few hours later. We would ask him a question and he would go into a long speech that made no sense.

At around 11 P.M., I called the emergency room and heard the fateful question, "Does anyone in his family have bipolar disorder?" I didn't really even know what the word was. Then the operator asked, "Does someone in his family have manic depression?" I said, "Wow! I think his father has that!" This is when his hospitalization started.

♦ Fears about financial problems due to reckless spending when manic or hypomanic or if your partner can't work. This is often the scariest part of loving someone with bipolar disorder.

♦ Hurt by things the ill person says during periods of intense irritability or dysphoric (agitated) manias. It's often shocking to hear what can come out of your partner's mouth when he or she gets sick. It can be hard to forgive.

♦ Embarrassment. It can be very difficult to face friends or family members if your partner does something embarrassing during an episode.

These problems illustrate what you may have experienced for a long time. You may be frustrated by the medication side effects that affect your partner's ability to function. He or she may sleep all day or have trouble sleeping at all. If your partner experiences weight gain, bad skin, and stomach problems, it's not exactly sexy! Another problem is that people with bipolar disorder are often irritable, frustrated, and impatient. They can get angry easily or pick on you incessantly. Impulsive manic behavior can lead to financial, legal, and work problems. Depression can make your once-vibrant partner shut down completely, and arguments often arise due to your confusion as to why this stuff is happening! In the past, before you read this book or consulted other sources, you may not have known this was all normal. You may have said the following to your partner:

♦ Why don't you just try harder?

♦ You would get better if you really loved me!

♦ What about the children? How can you ignore the children like this?

♦ You did *what*?

Along with the above questions, you may have experienced the following thoughts:

♦ We never have sex and to tell the truth, you're not really sexy anymore.

♦ You shut me out.

♦ I'm scared you'll kill yourself.

♦ The mania is taking all of our money.

♦ You can't work.

♦ We can't go anywhere.

♦ I worry you will be sick forever.

♦ If you stop your medications again, I'm leaving.

♦ This illness costs too much.

♦ You do things I know make you ill.

♦ I want to leave when you get really ill.

♦ I feel like the illness is taking over our lives.

♦ I want children, but I don't want them to have this illness.

- We never really talk anymore.

- I'm tired of taking care of you.

- I love you so much and don't know what to do next.

- I get frustrated when you're so slow.

- I'm scared you will have an affair when manic.

- I work and you don't yet you don't keep the house clean.

- When I want to talk, you get silent, and I hate that.

- I want to help you, but I have no idea how to help you!

That is a lot for one person to deal with. I went through all of these when Ivan was sick and I know he went through similar thoughts living with my undiagnosed bipolar disorder. It's normal if you regularly deal with these thoughts and feelings. Bipolar disorder creates a lot of chaos and often makes it impossible for you to know what is real and what is a result of your partner's mood swings. As you treat bipolar disorder more effectively, you may find that many items on the preceding list get better or go away completely. And even more important, if you and your partner can create an environment where good communication is stressed, you can go over the list together and talk about your feelings. Now that you have a better idea of what your partner goes through and know that your reactions to his or her behavior are normal, it's time for you both to learn how to treat bipolar disorder first.

Treat Bipolar Disorder First

Successful couples know that treating this illness is paramount. Managing the illness comes before you can have fun together, take trips, be great parents, and have a loving sex life. Treating bipolar disorder first comes before everything for one reason: when bipolar disorder isn't treated first, your entire life can be negatively affected by mood swings. If your partner goes on and off medications, gets manic once a year, or has been depressed for months, you know this. Many couples will go to therapy hoping to improve their relationship when managing the illness successfully may be all that's needed to see a great improvement. Then you can go to therapy to make things even better. Whew, isn't it great to know that managing the illness is often the solution to what you thought were relationship issues? I know it eases my mind. The next step is to think about yourself separately from your partner and the illness.

Safeguarding Your Health and Well-Being

Here is something "selfish" to consider: you come first in any relationship. Period. Without a healthy "you" there is no "us." It's hard to remember this when the person you care about has just tried to kill herself or the man you love screamed at you and wouldn't leave the house. Luckily, there are steps you can take to make sure you come first so that you can be there in good times and bad. One way to do this is to get really clear on what you're like when you're not in a bipolar crisis. I call this finding your base mood. Once you know your base mood and then learn the base mood of your partner, you can use the information to distinguish whether the challenges you and your partner experience are typical relationship challenges or whether they are challenges caused by the illness. This is very important as organic relationship challenges are very, very different from the relationship "problems" you experience because of bipolar disorder.

Discover Your Base Mood

In the following exercise, you will rate the following statements on a scale of 1 to 10, with 1 being the positive number and 10 being the negative. You will use the first line, (a), for your numbers. The others will be used later.

Number your calmness when faced with a situation such as a child's bad grades, the loss of a promotion, or your partner's mood after he or she has a tough day.

a.____   b.____   c. ____   d. ____

Choose a number for your anger/irritation level when faced with the typical stresses we all face: traffic, difficult coworker, whiny child, etc.

a.____   b.____   c. ____   d. ____

Rate the love you feel for your partner when he or she is stable.

a.____   b.____   c. ____   d. ____

Write a number to describe your sexual feelings toward your partner when he or she is stable.

a.____   b.____   c. ____   d. ____

Rate the calmness with which you and your partner discuss life issues such as money, travel, sexuality, and communication when you are both stable.

a.____   b.____   c. ____   d. ____

Now, go back to the exercise and in blank (b) write the number you experience when your partner is ill. The first number is your base mood and the second is your mood when it's affected by bipolar disorder. This is very valuable information.

Discover Your Partner's Base Mood

It's important that just as with yourself, you know what your partner is like when he or she *isn't* in a mood swing. It's so easy to forget this information when you're in a crisis!

In column (c), choose a number to describe your partner in the situation when he or she is well. Then, in column (d), use a red pen and write a number that represents him or her when he or she is in a mood swing. It's even better if you and your partner can do this together.

Here's the secret. Learn and remember these numbers. When you find yourself going way beyond your baseline because of something in your relationship, there's a very good chance it's due to your partner's bipolar disorder. This is especially important to know if the numbers go off the charts suddenly—if your feelings for your stable partner are completely, 100 percent different when he or she cries during sex or doesn't come home from "work" until 2 A.M. when you know he or she would never have that behavior when stable. Knowing both of your base moods greatly increases your chance of treating bipolar disorder first. It's important to know what you're up against!

Real People

After we were both diagnosed, we floundered for years, especially regarding my bipolar disorder, as I had a lot of medication problems. After three years of this, in 1998, I realized that I had to change completely and treat this illness myself if I wanted us both to get well and have a vibrant relationship. I created the treatment plan I talk about in my books and made changes.

The main change I made was learning what was real and what was the illness. I learned that when Ivan was at his baseline mood, he had few problems with work, but when he started to get ill, he felt that his work was falling apart. I learned to recognize this and simply said, "Ivan, you always worry about work when you get sick. This is about bipolar disorder. Let's focus on treating the illness instead of what you feel is wrong with your work." This helped immensely and changed our relationship for the better. When I said things such as, "I don't have any friends," he would say, "Julie, you always say this when you get depressed. Are you feeling down today?" Then we could focus on what was really wrong. I was depressed. Wow, what a difference this made in our relationship!

Unreality	Reality
Nothing will get better.	Things definitely can get better.
Medications are enough.	Medications are important, but they are only a part of a treatment plan.
My partner will never want sex again.	Sexual desire comes back when the illness is treated successfully.
The side effects will last forever.	Medication side effects often improve over time.
Our relationship is doomed.	Relationships can actually improve when a couple faces a crisis together.
We can't have kids.	Many people have children when one partner has bipolar disorder.

Examining Your Expectations and Setting Your Limitations

As with any potentially difficult situation—and I say "potentially difficult" as it is very possible to live pleasurably, successfully, and joyfully with someone who has managed his or her bipolar disorder—it's up to you to learn as much as you can about the illness through the content of this book and other resources and then make decisions that keep *you* stable. This means you have to become a student of this illness and once you have more information, you have to ask yourself the question: what are my limits and what limits do I have to put on this relationship in order to keep us both happy? Coming up with an answer to this question is hard and may take a long time, but it's possible. The first step is to examine the expectations you had when you came into this relationship.

Here is an expectations list that may sound familiar:

- We will love and take care of each other.

- He/she will be my companion and partner during the big decisions of life.

- We will have great sex forever!

- We will work as a team.

- Of course, there will be problems and struggles, but we will face them together.

- He/she will be the same person I married.

Couples where bipolar disorder is *not* an issue can work toward these expectations through partnership, personal work, education, patience, and love. It's natural there will be rough times, but with work, life can be good and stable!

It can be the same when bipolar disorder is in the picture, but believe me, it's a lot more difficult. I could lie and tell you that things will be fine and that love can keep a couple going, but this is simply not the case. One major manic episode can wipe out every expectation on the preceding list. Or the realization that your partner can't work full time if he wants to stay stable can be a huge blow to any relationship.

If something catastrophic has already happened to you and you're working on repairing your relationship, there is a lot of hope. Ivan and I consciously and successfully discussed and repaired what happened during his mania and the months after: the affair, the fight on the train track, his extreme need for help when he came home from the hospital, and finally his inability to work for almost a year. I realized that my expectations would have to change. He was worth it and our relationship was stronger for what happened.

Real People

When I got sick a year after Ivan was diagnosed, I told him I didn't love him anymore, got on a plane, and went to China. I got sick in Hong Kong and went to Hawaii where my mom was living. I was put on antidepressants—a huge mistake—got manic, and went back to Ivan and said, "I'm cured!" I was finally diagnosed with Bipolar II—everyone thought I was just depressed and alternatively crazy, which is why my illness had been misdiagnosed for 15 years. No one talked much about hypomania back then! After all of this, Ivan was there for me in the same way I had been there for him. I had trouble working for years and he supported me. It was not what either of us wanted, but because we both made a commitment to manage the illness, we survived quite well!

Setting Limitations—Even When It's Painful!

This is going to be a short paragraph simply because only you know your limitations. I have friends who have extremely high tolerance levels when it comes to bipolar disorder behavior, while others simply won't be around someone with the illness.

Guilt from Setting Limitations Is Normal

These limitations can be so hard when you truly love someone and want to be with them. You can have huge feelings of guilt when you really start to take care of yourself by setting these limitations. You may think: "If I get tough and talk about my feelings, what will happen to my partner? Who will take care of him? What if he tries to kill himself? How will she respond when I tell her that I can't stay unless she takes her medications? How will this affect our children?"

Just as your partner's decisions have consequences when he or she is well, your decisions will have consequences. You have to decide the consequences you can handle. I suggest that you start with easy to accomplish requests regarding your limitations. Believe me, it can be a challenge if you have to say these things when the person you love is already under a lot of stress. But at some point, you have to come first. This is what makes a relationship strong.

Setting Limitations: What To Say

"I care about you and love you very much. I'm in this relationship because I feel we can have something wonderful together. When you don't manage your bipolar disorder, I doubt my ability to maintain my health and well-being. I want to let you know that when you do all you can to manage the illness, I will be there for you, because I know you're trying to help yourself. I understand what bipolar disorder does to you. But I also know that you can learn to manage the illness. I need you to do this every day. We can have an equal partnership when we work together."

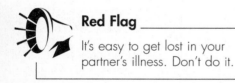

Red Flag

It's easy to get lost in your partner's illness. Don't do it.

Caretakers Beware!

Caretaking is the negative buzzword when you love someone with bipolar disorder. It's a fact that you will have to find a way to help your partner without being a caretaker. It's not an easy thing to do. People will say, be careful! You don't want to lose yourself in this illness. But they don't really have any idea what it's like to love and want to help a person with severe mood swings.

There are books on the caretaking topic now that we are more open about Alzheimer's disease and other physical illnesses that can't be treated by the individual alone. People tend to understand the challenges faced when you love someone with a brain tumor or Alzheimer's. The challenge you face with bipolar disorder is that people may not see that you need help. Your partner may seemingly look fine, go to work every day, and have fun with friends. But when your partner falls apart, you are the one who's there when the fun stops and the person you care about can't get out of bed.

Caretaking is a complicated topic. Here's a definition that can help:

caretaking   Losing yourself in the care of another person. Changing your life to care for the other person. Worrying day and night about the other person. Stopping what once gave you pleasure to care for the other person. Explaining away inappropriate behavior, especially violence, because you're embarrassed by the other person. When you get down to the basics, caretaking means you're doing more than you would normally to make sure your partner is okay physically and mentally and you lose yourself in the process. When things are unequal like this for too long, relationships can suffer.

Hmm. Does this sound familiar?

Caretaking turns into enabling when you don't set limits that protect you from your partner's behavior. Enabling means you let your partner stay in bed for weeks while you take care of the house, or you ignore the signs that your partner is getting manic and lie to his or her boss when he or she raises concerns. Enabling is covering up bipolar disorder behavior that needs to be treated and changed.

Real People

I was the ultimate caretaker when Ivan was in the hospital and I now regret it. I did what I thought was natural. I stopped my life and took care of him 24 hours a day until he was better. Of course, some people helped, but the burden and especially the debilitating worry were with me the entire time. We had just moved to the States and I lost my job. I didn't make new friends and I spent hours writing in my journal because I missed him so much when he was in the hospital. I had to go to the hospital every day because he refused meds unless I was there and I had to deal with all of the doctors. How on Earth was I supposed to take care of myself when he needed so much care?

This was more than 10 years ago, when there wasn't much talk about partners and what we go through. It would be very, very different now if Ivan got sick, because I know how to help without being a caretaker. You can learn to do the same.

Take Care of Yourself Today

Let's get this out of the way: if your partner has had mood swings in the past with serious consequences or currently has untreated bipolar disorder, you have to protect yourself physically, emotionally, and as a parent. Here are some tips on how to take care of yourself today so that you can be there for your partner tomorrow.

Physically

Adrenaline runs high when someone you love is sick and possibly in danger, and too much adrenaline can make *you* very stressed and anxious. Stress can skyrocket a hormone called cortisol, which can seriously affect your immune system and make you more susceptible to illnesses. I was once so scared that Ivan was actually going to kill himself, I almost passed out. You may drive under this stress and have an accident. And there is a good chance that your appetite and exercise schedule can really get thrown off when you're in a bipolar disorder crisis. And finally, sleep can be seriously affected, which is always a detriment to your health.

◆ Exercise every day, no matter what. It's especially helpful to do this with an understanding friend.

◆ Don't eat like a monster or starve yourself from the stress. I've found that sugar really isn't a cure for my partner's mood swings!

◆ Take sleep meds if you need them. Talk with your doctor about this.

Emotionally

Everyone responds differently to a bipolar crisis. You may shut off your emotions and not ask for help. Others may reach out too much and become overly needy. You can become depressed or so stressed you yell at your children and your partner! Luckily, this is an area where there is a lot of outside help available.

◆ Find a therapist who has experience with caretaking.

◆ Ask around and find someone who has experienced and survived the illness of a partner and ask for their guidance.

◆ Seek spiritual help if that works for you.

◆ Be very honest about your emotions.

As a Parent

Children have to be protected from out-of-control bipolar disorder behavior at all times. When your children are old enough—even as early as 5 or 6 years old—you can explain what is happening in an appropriate way. For example, "You know how Mama gets sick and sometimes cries all day and can't make your lunch? This is because she has an illness called bipolar disorder. It can be treated and we can work together to help her. There is no reason to be scared—things are being taken care of."

I've told my nephew about my mood swings from the time he was old enough to talk. At first I would say, "Auntie Wee is sick today." When he was older, I explained depression. It helps to ask questions such as "David, have you ever noticed that I have days where I can't play or talk as much as usual?" This made it a lot easier for me to spend time with him.

You can definitely explain bipolar disorder to your children without scaring them or making a big deal out of the illness. It's better than keeping secrets and upsetting the child when your partner changes moods. Being honest with your children when appropriate is a huge relief and helps you focus on them instead of always being a caretaker.

- ◆ Talk with a child psychologist before talking with your child.

- ◆ Ask for advice from your teenagers. They are often much more observant than you think.

- ◆ Involve grandparents and tell them exactly what you need.

Taking care of yourself physically, emotionally, and as a parent covers all of the bases and helps you remain stable even when your partner is not.

Finances: Show Me the Money!

This warrants a separate section, as money is almost always an issue with bipolar disorder. Mania makes people spend recklessly, and depression can affect a person's ability to work. Psychosis can make your partner make some very scary financial decisions. There is one solution to this problem that is going to be hard, but it works. *You have to take charge of the money in your relationship until your partner is stable enough to do it with you.* Ouch.

Finances: What to Say

"If you had a physical illness, we would make financial changes. Let's do the same now. Bipolar disorder takes away your reasoning ability—it's a completely normal symptom of the illness. I want to protect myself and you from this unreasonable thinking. Let's do it together. I have all of the bills, accounts, and other areas I think we need to discuss. I just want you to know this is no reflection on you or your strength—it's about bipolar disorder and our financial future."

Real People

When Ivan, who didn't have spending problems with his mania, said he no longer wanted my name on our investments, I was pretty devastated. I did have a history of spending when I was manic and it was the right decision, but it hurt! I understood that we should have separate accounts in all that we did. Truthfully, this was not a big issue, as I was unable to earn much money at the time! That alone was embarrassing and sad.

Many years later, this is no longer a problem. I've learned to control my mania to the point that I rarely have manic spending disasters, but at the time it was essential. I learned that the financial decisions we had to make at the beginning changed completely once I managed the illness. These changes were not set in stone.

Getting Clear on Your Finances

You will need information, including account numbers and passwords, for the following:

◆ Bank accounts

◆ Credit cards

◆ Insurance policies

◆ Retirement funds

Red Flag

Getting realistic about the effects of bipolar disorder on finances can be embarrassing, shameful, and for a man, emasculating. Be gentle and tread lightly when you talk about the issues.

Considering that love is not a treatment for bipolar disorder, you have to take care of the above no matter how much it hurts. When your partner is stable, you can discuss a financial power of attorney and you can definitely ask your partner for advice on how to protect you from his or her mood swings. Your partner doesn't want to hurt you financially. He or she may readily agree to have all of the above in your name until the illness has been stabilized for a few years.

Know Your Legal Rights as a Partner

What happened to me may be familiar to you, but it doesn't have to happen again in the future. You can visit the National Alliance on Mental Illness (NAMI) at www.nami.org or the Depression and Bipolar Support Alliance (DBSA) at www.dbsa.org to find out your legal rights depending on where you live.

> **Real People** _____
>
> It's not a secret that I believe we have gone too far with patient rights in this country. Laws in many states require the permission of the person who is ill in order for you to get much-needed information. This often isn't possible when your partner is no longer coherent mentally. When Ivan was in the hospital there wasn't as much restriction on information as there is now, but I was still pretty much ignored when it came to whether he could stay in the hospital.
>
> After he had been in the hospital for two months, I had to go to court to get Ivan more help. He was appointed an attorney. Ivan arrived in a wheelchair and was strapped down because he was so agitated and psychotic. It broke my heart to see him: We all sat down and the attorney started to argue for Ivan's rights. The judge then looked at Ivan and said, "Do you feel you need to be in the hospital?" Ivan said, "No," and I felt like screaming. Then the judge asked one more time and Ivan looked around and said, "Has Julie been shot?" They let him back into the hospital.
>
> Things have not gotten much better. These days, even if your partner is so psychotic he can't talk, you have even less access to his or her treatment.

Prepare for the Future While Your Partner Is Stable

The best time to implement the suggestions in this chapter is when your partner is stable. You can then be very open about how these changes make both of you feel. Despite how sexist this may sound, the limitations caused by bipolar disorder can be especially hard for men who were raised to take care of their families or for women who want to have children even though they are on medications. It's very important to note that a person just out of the hospital or someone coming down from a manic high or returning from a suicidal low needs time to recover. This is not the time to discuss the ideas in this chapter, but you can do them alone. So many couples, without the stresses of a mental illness, never discuss the important issues that adversely affect a relationship. Although I know that bipolar disorder is not a positive, talking about the issues you face because of the illness can be an incredibly bonding experience.

Conclusion

Untreated bipolar disorder is not okay. It puts too much pressure on the family, especially children, and makes it pretty impossible for you to have a relationship with the person you love. Luckily, management is not as difficult as it may seem—especially if you're reading this right after your partner was diagnosed. I got better and Ivan got better.

It's so true that couples who work together to keep bipolar disorder in check can have relationships that are more open and loving than those around them. It takes courage to be this honest with each other, but the rewards are better communication and a deeper understanding of what you and your partner are capable of. Having a common cause and goal—to have a successful relationship even though one partner has bipolar disorder—can unite a family and create an unbreakable bond between the two of you. The result can be a very successful, companionable, honest, and open relationship. It's true, something positive really can happen when someone you love has bipolar disorder!

The Least You Need to Know

- ◆ It's normal to be completely overwhelmed and scared when your partner is diagnosed with bipolar disorder.

- ◆ You don't have to become a caretaker and get lost in your partner's illness. You can learn to help without caretaking.

- ◆ It's essential that you and your family are protected from financial disasters caused by bipolar disorder.

- ◆ Couples who work together to manage bipolar disorder can be the envy of all of their friends, simply because they have such great communication skills! This can be true for you!

Chapter 23

For Parents of a Bipolar Preteen or Young Teen

In This Chapter

- ◆ Typical bipolar teen problems
- ◆ How to best help your child
- ◆ A second opinion from Dr. Gransee

Parenting any teen or preteen can have its share of challenges. When you add bipolar disorder to the mix, it's enough to make even the most patient parent want to scream. In this chapter, we'll share some tips and information especially directed toward parents of young people with bipolar disorder.

What to Expect

Expect the unexpected. That should be the mantra of every parent with a bipolar child, especially once the child hits the preteen and teenage years. We wish we could give you an exact blueprint of how your child will act and when. Unfortunately, it's not that simple.

Bipolar disorder can be unpredictable, even in adults. With younger people, that unpredictability is much greater, partly because of all of the chemical and hormonal changes the child is going through due to puberty and normal growth. So having a bipolar teen is kind of like riding a roller coaster with lots of blind curves. You never know what you're gonna get next, but it won't be as good as a box of chocolates. However, here are a few general things you're likely to encounter.

Extreme Mood Swings

Obviously, a bipolar person of any age has a tendency to go through mood swings. With young people, however, these mood swings can often come on more suddenly—and fluctuate more rapidly—because of all the chemicals and hormones going at full speed inside their brains.

Social Difficulties

The teenage years are tough on everyone, what with peer pressure, school issues, trying to fit in, and so on. Bipolar teens have it especially tough, because they often have trouble making friends easily. In addition, if they've had any kind of "strange" episodes in school or need to take medication in school—or worse, miss school due to a hospitalization—they may be targets for taunts and teasing from other kids.

The problem is, this can often make the teen want to withdraw and isolate himself—which, as you know, can spell big trouble for someone who is bipolar. Many bipolar kids find it works best to hang out with a small, close-knit group of kids, or maybe even just one or two really close friends. These good friends are less likely to judge or tease the bipolar teen.

If you can help your child establish a few good friendships, it can make a world of difference. You also want to help him keep the friends he already has. This may mean educating those kids on bipolar disorder and its symptoms, so they won't hold your child's moods and other symptoms against him.

Medication Problems

As if your bipolar teen didn't have enough problems already, you may discover that his meds—the ones that have been working like a charm until this point—suddenly don't work. Or worse, they may start causing new side effects. This isn't unusual. Some bipolar meds that work well for adults aren't recommended for kids, whereas other meds that work fine for a child may not address a bipolar adult's needs. The hormonal and chemical changes associated with puberty can affect how medications work for your child.

Red Flag

If you notice any change in how your child is reacting to his meds, especially if any new side effects appear, be sure to alert the doctor right away.

A Big Improvement (If You're Lucky)

Occasionally bipolar children will be completely transformed during the teenage years. Sometimes they show great improvement in their moods and behavior, and they may even make such strides that they are able to be weaned off their meds.

This could be due to a number of things. First, it's possible that the child wasn't really bipolar at all, and was simply misdiagnosed. There's also the possibility that the chemical changes in the brain during puberty somehow triggered a reaction that "adjusted" the child's system. Some parents believe that their child "grew out" of bipolar disorder, although that isn't technically possible.

What is likely is that a child who shows dramatic improvement is flying under the radar for bipolar disorder. The genetics aren't acting up and the bipolar monster has gone to sleep. Hopefully the monster will stay asleep. There are preventative measures to take to make sure he doesn't wake up.

Whatever the reason, if you're one of the relatively few lucky parents blessed with this unexpected surprise, enjoy it!

How to Help Your Child

Your support and encouragement are invaluable to your bipolar child, even if he or she may not always seem to welcome your help. It's like the little boy who doesn't want his friends to see his mom kiss him goodbye when she drops him off at school. Secretly, he is happy she tried, and he might be upset if she didn't.

Here are some ways you can make things easier for your child:

◆ **Talk.** Keep the lines of communication open. Don't be too pushy, but let your child know you're always available if he or she needs to talk.

◆ **Educate and empower.** Teens like to feel independent and powerful. Give your teen as much information as possible about bipolar disorder, and be sure to let him or her take an active role in decisions related to treatment.

◆ **Give your child some space.** Teens like to have their privacy, and bipolar teens are no different. If you're constantly hovering and butting in, that will just make it more difficult for your child to have a normal social life.

◆ **Pay attention.** Give your child space, but stay alert for any signs of trouble. By nipping a problem in the bud early on, you can spare your child from experiencing a major episode.

Becoming an Advocate for Your Child

While your bipolar teen may feel like an adult, the truth is that he or she is still a minor and can only do so much alone. You can serve a valuable role as your child's advocate, making sure she gets the help she needs.

You might need to deal with teachers and school administrators to ensure your child is getting any special services she requires. You want to take a team approach, enlisting their help in making your child's school experience the best it can be.

Mental Note

As your bipolar child's advocate (and legal decision maker), you may need to navigate lots of bureaucratic red tape: insurance forms, school paperwork, and the like. Do your research to make sure you fully understand everything. It can be helpful to join support groups or online forums, where you can get answers and advice from other parents who have already handled these issues.

In addition, you'll be your child's advocate when it comes to treatment decisions. This is a tricky area. Your child is now old enough to actively participate in her treatment—and decisions affecting it—but she isn't legally entitled to make her own decisions. Technically, as the parent, you can make the decisions for your child. But things will go much more smoothly if you and your child are in agreement about the best treatment options.

You may also need to serve as your child's representative when it comes to legal or bureaucratic matters—dealing with insurance companies, for example.

Impact on the Family

As we've said before, bipolar disorder doesn't just affect the person who has it. The entire family feels the impact, and this is especially true when it's a young person who has BP. Having a bipolar teen in the house can be stressful, challenging, and exhausting for the parents as well as any other siblings. Just dealing with all of the appointments, school meetings, and other obligations can seem like a full-time job.

Here are some things you can do to lessen the negative impact on your family:

- **Participate in family counseling.** This allows everyone to express their feelings and frustrations in a safe environment. Plus, the therapist can teach you ways to better handle stressful situations related to the bipolar child.

- **Don't let bipolar disorder rule your family.** This isn't always possible, especially if your child is experiencing a period of major symptoms. But as much as possible, you want to enjoy normal family activities and experiences.

- **Pay attention to other siblings.** It can be tough to be the brother or sister of a bipolar teen. Your other kids may start to feel left out if all of your attention is focused on the bipolar child. It won't always be easy to juggle everything (and everyone), but try your best to give your other children enough one-on-one attention.

Dr. Gransee Weighs In

Dr. Jonathan Gransee is a psychologist specializing in evaluations for disability determination and other purposes. In the next few sections, he shares his observations and opinions related to bipolar disorder in young people.

The current trend is leaning toward more diagnoses of BP in children and the use of medication as the primary treatment. Dr. Gransee takes a conservative approach in the use of medication and the diagnosis of bipolar disorder in children. We wanted to include as many different views and voices as possible, and we think Dr. Gransee's thoughts are worth pondering.

The Soaring Diagnosis Rate

Most treatment professionals working with children and adolescents are acutely aware of the rise in the rate at which children and adolescents, but most significantly prepubescent children, are being diagnosed with bipolar disorder.

While estimates vary, it is interesting to note several recently reported statistics. *The New York Times,* in an article published in September 2007, noted that in the 10-year span from 1993 to 2003, there was a 40-fold increase in the rate at which the child and adolescent population was being diagnosed with bipolar disorder, while a more scholarly article (Youngstrom, 2005) noted that marked increases had been found in the rate of diagnosis in children involved with Child Protective Services in Illinois.

Other writers have pointed to this sharp increase in the rate, some approvingly (*The New York Times,* 2007; Papolos and Papolos, 2006), saying that even more of an increase is needed. Others, however, have expressed alarm at this sharp increase, pleading with professionals to take a more conservative approach toward diagnosing BP in young people.

There is much debate and contention brought on by the huge gulf between the most liberal and the most conservative views on this issue. To some extent, this divide is evident between psychiatrists and psychologists, and indeed, the previously noted *New York Times* article pointed out that 90 percent of the diagnosing of bipolar disorder in children was being done by psychiatrists. However, there are many other mental health professionals, including psychologists and other non-psychiatric folk in the field, who take the liberal approach.

What's Behind the Increase?

For those who advocate earlier diagnosis, one of the most commonly cited reasons is prevention: prevention of a poor childhood, prevention of academic difficulties, prevention of social failure, prevention of kindling, and so on. The risk, proponents of earlier diagnosis believe, is that failure to act is a disservice to the child and to those involved in the child's life.

This has been the reasoning driving such professionals as Dr. Demitri Papolos, his wife Janice Papolos, and others—indeed, any professional with a modicum of empathy has considered this when reflecting on a possible case of bipolar disorder in a child or adolescent. If allowing children to pass through childhood without appropriate treatment sentences them to a substandard future, who among us would hesitate to act? The problem is that it is not entirely clear that we have gotten this right, and it is certainly not clear that what appears to be bipolar disorder in a child will follow the child into adulthood.

The Conservative Approach

The conservative approach toward diagnosing bipolar disorder in children is to keep the status quo. In other words, the child or adolescent must meet the criteria for major depression and for mania in terms of severity of symptoms and duration of the moods. In this approach, the child would need to show severe depression for a week, in most cases, and would have to show chronic mania for the better part of a week, before he or she could be considered for the diagnosis. In instances in which there was thought to be a mixed episode, these duration criteria could be waived, but the severity criteria could not.

The Liberal Approach

The more liberal approaches vary, but there is a general relaxation of the duration and frequency criteria, to the point that, in the most liberal approach, children can cycle from minute to minute! The more liberal approach also tends to redefine what comprises depression or mania in children, with the most liberal approach defining mania as consisting primarily of chronic and severe irritation or general anger issues. Depression, in this approach, may primarily manifest as anger or social withdrawal.

Interim Conclusion

The problem with the conservative approach, in some professionals' views, is that we are potentially missing children who should have a BP diagnosis and treatment. And indeed, when a child or adolescent has significant emotional or behavioral issues that go untreated, his life does often go from bad to worse.

The problem with the liberal approach is that treatment, which is led by the medical approach, involves the introduction of potentially toxic psychotropics into the child's body. Most of the psychotropics used to treat bipolar disorder in children and adolescents are prescribed "off-label," without the sanctioning of the FDA, and without knowledge of the potential long-term side effects of such treatment on the developing body and brain.

Current Research

Because of the saliency of this particular area of mental health, there has been a great deal of research on this topic in the past decade or longer. The National Institute of

Mental Health (NIMH), the National Alliance on Mental Illness (NAMI), and other organizations have funded multiple studies to answer questions related to this debate. Books have been written on this, including *The Bipolar Child* (Papolos and Papolos, 2006, and earlier editions). So what is the state of the science? What do we know?

According to Papolos and Papolos, in an informal research study that involved polling parents who had identified their children as bipolar, there was a great deal of diversity in what symptoms might be seen in a child or adolescent with bipolar disorder. Papolos and Papolos identified moodiness, nightmares, sleep problems, sensory integration difficulties, extreme temper tantrums, depression, food sensitivities, anxiety, hyperactivity, impulsivity, distractibility, oppositional behavior, and other traits. Indeed, they were of the mind that because bipolar disorder spanned such an array of symptoms (many of which were found in other childhood mental disorders, such as autism, Asperger's syndrome, oppositional defiant disorder, attention-deficit hyperactivity disorder, post-traumatic stress disorder, and the like), one should diagnose the BP disorder first, and then consider additional diagnoses if the symptoms were not fully explained by the first diagnosis.

While Papolos and Papolos's conclusions were by far the most extreme, many researchers feel that a much more liberal interpretation of what bipolar disorder is in children is needed. The consensus seems to be that children with bipolar disorder will not meet the same measures of frequency and duration required for diagnosis in adulthood.

Most liberal diagnosticians maintain that children and young adolescents can "cycle daily," that they may not demonstrate traditional mania, and that their depression may not necessarily be debilitating. Most liberal diagnosticians also maintain that irritability may be part of mania and that bipolar children seem to have severe anger problems. Questions that have not been definitively answered center around differential diagnoses. (For example, is it bipolar disorder, or post-traumatic stress disorder, or both?)

What If the Liberal Approach Is Right?

If the liberal approach holds up to the scrutiny of time and research, then there are many children who have rightly been provided with attention and treatment that may prevent future problems. Such a proactive approach may improve public opinion of the mental health field, as well, and may increase funding directed toward mental health problems or insurance company recognition of mental health problems.

What If the Conservative Approach Is Right?

If the conservatives are right, then we potentially have a public disaster on our hands. Treatment of children and young adolescents with bipolar medications is unproven, sometimes (or often) ineffective, and marred by the many side effects and potential long-term damage. Bipolar medications can cause agitation; increased behavioral difficulty; moodiness; weight gain; shaking; tiredness; and potentially more serious problems, such as polycystic ovarian syndrome, or a sometimes deadly skin disease; tremors; seizures; and death.

As well, it may be that telling a child that she has less control over her emotions and behaviors than a typical child could cause her to give up and to actually worsen in her behaviors. Also, some suggest that medicating children at a young age imbues in them a belief that substances are the answer for their ills … and how far down the road from that is the belief that illicit substances may be the answer?

How Well Are We Doing?

Given all the concerns, how are we doing? What do we know about the effectiveness of the more liberal diagnostic approach? Reviewing the literature, the results are not encouraging. For instance, Dr. John March of Duke University points out that we have no idea whether children diagnosed between the ages of 5 to 7 will actually be bipolar when they are older.

The New York Times article previously cited notes that most research suggests that these kids are more likely to have depression, rather than bipolar disorder, as they get older. Generally, it appears that medications often do not address the bulk of the symptoms, and their strongest effect seems to be in the sedation category, which is a double-edged sword. Specifically, the child or young adolescent becomes more manageable and less volatile, but he or she is also sometimes less able to focus on academics, and he or she may experience major personality shifts, with undesirable effects on his or her social success.

Mood stabilization is often an elusive goal, even with heavy psychopharmacological intervention, and in some instances, the patient's mood becomes more unstable during pharmacological treatment. The side effects often become an issue in and of themselves, necessitating additional medications, diet changes, new academic approaches, and even adjustments in general expectations of the child's ability to function. In some instances, the medications make the child potentially eligible for disability benefits, because of the debilitating effects they have on the child's functioning.

As well, in many instances the pharmacological interventions are being guided by overworked and overwhelmed child and adolescent psychiatrists, who cannot spend the time needed to fully evaluate children and their needs. They are often pressured by pharmacological companies, directly and indirectly, to prescribe particular medications or to identify a certain portion of their caseloads as bipolar. Even if one accepts the thinking that bipolar disorder in children and adolescents is underdiagnosed, and that bipolar children should be treated with medications, the end result is often partial or full failure to address the issue.

Are We Missing Something?

Research completed by Martin Teicher, M.D., Ph.D. (2000) suggests that early trauma, be it sexual, physical, or verbal, has a potentially long-term effect on the developing brain. His research indicates that such trauma, and particularly verbal abuse, causes long-term changes in the corpus callosum and in the hypothalamus, as well as in other areas. The corpus callosum is important in balancing the right and left brains, and those with underdeveloped corpus callosi tend to be very reactive or unbalanced in their approaches to problem solving (that is, they are overly emotional and emotionally reactive … in other words, more likely to be angry, violent, or irrational).

Those with this pattern of brain misdevelopment tend to be less logical, less integrated in their personalities, and generally inappropriate in their reactions. Thus, in Teicher's view, many of the behavioral and mood issues that we see in prepubescent or postpubescent children may be a result of those early childhood experiences.

In other words, Teicher is proving something clinicians on the front lines have thought all along: subjecting a child to abuse tends to cause the child to experience major personality shifts, often causing the child to become violent and emotional. If Dr. Teicher prevails at the end of the day, it may well be that what we think is childhood bipolar disorder is actually a trauma disorder. And the implications of that are the difference between labeling a child as potentially temporarily impaired or permanently impaired.

Conclusion

There is much debate about the frequency with which childhood bipolar disorder occurs in children and adolescents. There is no questioning the conclusion that this is an important area to explore, as the implications for this disorder over the lifetime of a person are serious. However, we need to get it right, because if not, we will either have undiagnosed cases that permanently alter children's chances for success, or we will have overmedicated children struggling with the side effects of unnecessary medications. Ultimately, science should clear the air—good, logical, replicable science that will show us what bipolar disorder probably looks like, if it indeed exists, in children. Until we have a scientific consensus, however, caution seems advisable. The more conservative approach would be to consider other, less long-term explanations for a child's symptom set.

Specific Parenting Issues

Now that we've covered the general stuff about parenting a bipolar teen, we'd like to address some specific concerns and issues you'll probably face.

The Issue of Medication

Whether or not to use medication is a big issue in the treatment of a child with a mental health problem. Does the child have a physiological problem like bipolar disorder or a psychological problem such as post-traumatic stress disorder? Is the child being diagnosed correctly?

The first assumption is that the child does have a mental health problem. If the parents bring their child to a mental health professional who diagnoses a mental health problem or refers the child to a specialist, we can be pretty sure the child has a mental health problem. Otherwise the mental health professional may tell the parents the child is normal or the parents are overreacting or may look at the parents with a hairy eyeball and invite the parents to come in for therapy.

Let's assume the child has a mental health problem. Okay, what is it? Is it physiological in nature or psychological? Well, if you go to a medical doctor (psychiatrist), he is trained in physiological problems. A psychologist is trained in psychological problems. You may want to get opinions from both. If the diagnosis is bipolar disorder, that is physiological and genetic. There would almost have to be someone in the family who exhibited similar behavior or could have been diagnosed with bipolar disorder. Maybe it was Grandma, but we are not sure because she committed suicide at the age of 24. Maybe it was Grandpa, who drank a lot (self-medicating?) and was a womanizer (hypersexuality?).

In 6,000 evaluations that this author has done in his lifetime, he has never seen a "spontaneous" case of bipolar disorder. There has always been a family member somewhere who showed the behavioral signs and could have had the genetics. The things that *looked* like bipolar disorder without a family history turned out to be chronic Lyme disease, hyperthyroidism, or another disorder. In other cases of bipolar disorder where there was no family history, the child had been adopted. In one case, the mother of the child had been adopted. Family history can be the biggest clue as to whether a mental health problem is physical or psychological.

So let's say there seems to be a family history of bipolar disorder. We have done a Lyme titer test, tested the thyroid, and we don't see a substance abuse problem. Our best guess is that the child has bipolar disorder. The next question to ask is: what woke up the bipolar monster?

- The hormonal changes of adolescence? (Most likely.)

- A trauma?

- Family dysfunction?

- Drugs, illegal drugs, prescription drugs, or steroids?

- A recluse spider bite?

- Sleep deprivation?

- Significant time zone change? (For example, moving to the United States from overseas.)

If none of the above items apply, the child's case could be a genetic early onset of bipolar disorder, which is extremely rare, unless the biological mother used drugs while pregnant (illegal drugs, anesthesia, or other prescription drugs).

If this explanation doesn't make sense either, then maybe we should check for a psychological problem or a different diagnosis than bipolar disorder.

Let's suppose we are satisfied that the child could have bipolar disorder. Now what? Consider medication. In these times, medication is the primary method of treatment for bipolar disorder in children. Children are usually difficult to medicate, because they are changing. Their medication may work for a while, but often eventually has to be switched or added to. In any case, the child is usually treated and hopefully stabilized on medication. The dosing can be inexact for children, because their bodies are always growing and changing.

As we said before, bipolar gets exacerbated by other things. Otherwise it flies under the radar in most children. There may be some prodromal symptoms, like a mild to moderate depression that first appears before adolescence. If the child is young and a specific event has exacerbated the bipolar disorder (such as a divorce), maybe once the family upheaval has diminished and there is a routine again (the child sees Dad every Tuesday and every other weekend, for example), we should consider titrating the child off the medication slowly, hoping the child will again fly under the radar. This would involve a concerted effort with the therapist, parents, and doctor working together. If a trauma exacerbated the bipolar monster, maybe therapy could diminish or erase the trauma.

Like Dr. Gransee, this author believes that bipolar disorder may be overdiagnosed and medication may not be the only treatment. Research shows that psychotherapy (as an adjunct to medication) shows excellent results in the treatment of bipolar disorder. This author sees a need for medication, but on a temporary basis. If the child doesn't fly under the radar and therapy doesn't help, then yes, medication is perhaps the only other option.

Raising Bipolar Kids

I wish I had known my child had bipolar genetics and I wish that I had known what I know now. I would have raised her differently. I would have raised her to realize how important sleep was. When the other kids in college were staying up all night studying for an exam, she would have known she couldn't do that. It could dangerously exacerbate her BP. I would have raised her to know her limitations. I raised all my children to think that they could do *anything*. That was good for my children without bipolar disorder.

I am going to generalize about what I have learned about bipolar kids from the many parents in my seminars who have raised them, from a colleague who does seminars on bipolar kids, from special education teachers, from research, and from books on bipolar children that agree with the feedback of these experienced people. Not all bipolar kids will match these descriptions, but many do, and if your kid does, you'll be happy to have this information.

Temper Tantrums

Bipolar kids seem to have temper tantrums that last longer than half an hour (sometimes all afternoon). The normal length of a temper tantrum is usually 12 to 20 minutes—until the adrenaline runs out. Then the child is exhausted and may even fall asleep. Bipolar kids have temper tantrums that seem to be unstoppable. The normal kid or ADHD kid will have a temper tantrum because he didn't get his way or because his feelings were hurt. A bipolar kid has a temper tantrum because you interrupted his routine or his plan.

How can you diminish the temper tantrums? Never interrupt a bipolar child's plan or routine. After the first 20 minutes of a tantrum, if you notice, the child is no longer trying to get his way. He is on the wave of the tantrum and it is not willful. He wants to get off, but he can't, and he doesn't like it. I'll explain.

Routines

Having a routine seems to be one of the most important things in a bipolar kid's life.

A mother of a bipolar child went to pick up her child at school. She spoke to a couple teachers and said, "I don't know how you put up with my Johnny. He is such a tyrant at home." The teachers looked at each other and one said, "Oh, no. We love little Johnny. He isn't that way here." Then they looked at the mother suspiciously.

What was this mother doing wrong? You see, at school, Johnny knows what he is going to be doing every five minutes. There is a routine. Maybe Mom doesn't have a routine.

Here is an example of a routine:

1. When you get home from school, you can play with your friends.

2. We are eating dinner at 6:00 P.M.

3. After you eat, you have to do your homework.

4. When you finish your homework, you can watch TV or play on the computer or call your friends.

5. At 10:00 P.M., you have to get ready for bed.

6. At 10:15 P.M., you must be in bed.

I have heard a BP kid come up to his parent and say, "It's ten o'clock; you'd better tell me to go to bed."

Making Plans

To avoid a temper tantrum, you can teach your child to not make plans without checking with you. That will nip those temper tantrums before they happen.

If you tell little Johnny that you are going to pick him up after school at 3:00 P.M., you had better be there at 3:00 P.M., or you risk a temper tantrum. It's not a matter of dominance or not getting his way. It's simply that you said you would be there at 3:00. If you think you might be late, you should tell Johnny that you will pick him up between 3:00 and 3:15. He will be okay with that. If you are caught in a traffic jam and it gets to be 3:20, you are not going to like what you find in front of that school, or all the way home!

Bipolar kids are not "impossible." We just need to understand them.

Sexual Issues

Bipolar kids can be hypersexual. In the past, therapists have mistaken the hypersexuality for being eroticized, which is a sign that a child may have been sexually abused. BP kids may act inappropriately and appear seductive, but they don't know what they are doing. A child who has been sexually abused will do specific things, while a hypersexual child will be vague.

Bipolar kids and adults seem to respond well to physical touch. It seems to calm them down and create a bond. Just because your child may be hypersexual is no excuse not to touch him or her and show physical affection. In fact, it seems the more affectionate you are, the less hypersexual your child will be. Children are innocent. They do not know what they are doing. You may have to move a child or tell her to stop touching you in a certain area, but do not stop showing her appropriate physical affection.

The Least You Need to Know

- ◆ Parenting a bipolar child isn't easy, but keep in mind that your child is struggling with considerable challenges of his own.

- ◆ BP kids may be misunderstood. Don't assume the worst.

- ◆ BP kids are easier to manage when they have a routine. Any changes in a routine can set them off.

- ◆ BP kids usually respond well to and bond with physical affection.

- ◆ The decision to use medication may be necessary, but it should be well thought out.

Appendix A

Glossary

advance medical directive   Also known as an AMD or an advance directive, a legal document outlining how you would like to be treated should you be hospitalized for your mental condition.

amygdales   Structures in the temporal lobes that are involved in processing emotion, especially in the fear response.

anterior   A directional term meaning "toward the front of the brain." Anterior is the opposite of posterior.

Asperger's syndrome   Part of the autism spectrum of disorders, characterized by an inability or unwillingness to engage in normal social interaction.

association cortex   Located in the frontal, parietal, and temporal areas of the brain, they store long-term memories and help us draw connections in our knowledge and our experiences.

attention-deficit hyperactivity disorder   Also known as ADHD, this is a neurological developmental behavioral disorder which manifests as hyperactivity, distractibility, impulsivity, and forgetfulness.

bipolar disorder   A mental disorder characterized by extreme (and often sudden) mood swings.

borderline personality disorder   A disorder that can appear very similar to bipolar disorder but is psychologically based and often set off by post-traumatic stress disorder.

brainstem   Located just above the spinal cord, it includes three structures—the midbrain, medulla, and pons. The brainstem controls basic functions such as balance, breathing, and heart rate, as well as basic behaviors such as eating and copulating.

central nervous system   An all-inclusive name for the brain and the spinal cord.

central sulcus   A large inward fold in the brain tissue, running from the top to the middle of the brain. It marks the division between the frontal and parietal lobes.

cerebral cortex   The part of the brain that includes all four lobes—frontal, temporal, parietal, and occipital. The cortex carries out high-level functions such as attention, language, and memory, as well as mediating some bodily sensations and movements.

circadian rhythms   The patterns of physiological changes that accompany cycles of sleep and wakefulness.

clinical depression   A neurological chemical imbalance that may cause bouts of prolonged sadness, crying spells, changes in appetite and sleep patterns, irritability, anger, worry, anxiety, or other symptoms.

clinical social workers   Counselors who have completed a Master's degree in social work from an accredited graduate program and are qualified to render diagnoses and provide individual and group counseling.

comorbidity   Term used to indicate that a patient has another disease or condition, in addition to bipolar disorder (or whatever their primary problem is).

computerized tomography   Researchers use CT scans to create an image of the brain. CT scans are useful for revealing damaged or abnormal areas in the brain.

Diagnostic and Statistical Manual of Mental Disorders   Also known as the DSM, this manual is published by the American Psychiatric Association and lists diagnostic criteria for all mental health disorders.

diencephalon   A subcortical structure that is made up of the thalamus and the hypothalamus.

electroencephalograph   Also known as an EEG, this technology measures electrical activity in local areas of the brain. Because neurons use electricity to communicate, an EEG gives a decent measurement of levels of overall activity in particular areas of the brain.

forebrain   The part of the brain that involves categorization of concrete and conscious experiences, feelings, and thoughts.

frontal lobe   The most anterior area of the brain, located anterior to the central sulcus and superior to the lateral fissure. It controls many high-level functions, including planning, inhibition, and memory encoding. The primary motor cortex and prefrontal cortex are located in the frontal lobe.

functional magnetic resonance imaging   Also known as fMRI, researchers use this to take three-dimensional pictures of the brain at work. By studying the blood flow in the brain while a subject performs a particular task, researchers can discover which areas of the brain are being used.

Gage, Phineas   A nineteenth-century construction worker whose frontal lobe was destroyed in an accident, leaving the rest of his brain intact. His case has been widely studied to try to discover the functions of the frontal lobe.

gyrus   Outward folds in the surface of the brain's tissue.

Hebb's rule   "Cells that fire together, wire together," succinctly states the governing principle of long-term potentiation. If two neurons are repeatedly activated at the same time, the connection between them will be strengthened so that they can activate each other in the future.

hemisphere   The cortex of the brain is divided into a right and a left hemisphere, which appear to be mirror images of each other. The two hemispheres are almost entirely separate, connected only by a thick bundle of nerves called the corpus collosum.

hindbrain   Part of the brain comprised of the brainstem and cerebellum.

hippocampus   Located in the temporal lobe, this is responsible for the formation of new memories.

hormones   Chemicals in the bloodstream that act on various organs to adjust the body's vital physiological systems.

hypothalamus   Part of the diencephalon; responsible for hormone secretion in the body.

inferior   Directional term meaning "toward the bottom of the brain." Inferior is the opposite of superior.

inhibition   The ability to suppress one's initial reaction or inclination in favor of the correct choice. Inhibition is thought to be mediated by the frontal lobe.

licensed professional counselors   Counselors who have completed a Master's degree in psychology or counseling.

limbic system   The part of the brain consisting of the thalamus, hypothalamus, and amygdala. Together they monitor all of your internal organs and control your pituitary gland.

lobe   The cerebral cortex is divided into four sections, called lobes, along the lines of several major fissures and sulci. The four lobes are frontal, temporal, parietal, and occipital. Because there are two hemispheres in the brain, there are actually two of each lobe, one on the right and one on the left.

magnetic resonance imaging   Also known as MRI, researchers use this to take three-dimensional pictures of the brain at rest. By measuring water density, it can detect injured areas of the brain in a noninvasive way (no need to pry open the skull or even inject patients with anything).

mania   Uncontrolled—and often unreasonable—excitement, hyperactivity, or anger. In a bipolar person, it is often accompanied by feelings of superiority and invincibility.

medulla   The most inferior of three structures in the brainstem. It works together with the pons to control postural and vital reflexes.

midbrain   The most superior of three structures in the brainstem. It governs basic behaviors like eating and walking, and it works together with the pons to regulate levels of sleep and arousal.

motor neuron   These carry signals from the brain and spinal cord to the muscles and glands of the body.

nurse psychotherapists   Registered nurses who are trained in psychiatric care and mental health nursing.

occipital lobe   Located in the most posterior section of the brain, it deals mostly with visual information. The primary visual cortex is part of the occipital lobe.

parasympathetic system   Part of the autonomic system that controls bodily functions that promote growth, energy conservation, and regeneration.

parietal lobe   This contains the somatic sensory cortex and some association cortex.

peripheral nervous system   Includes sensory neurons and motor neurons. The components of the PNS dealing with motor neurons can be divided into the autonomic and the somatic systems.

plastic   Term used to describe areas of the brain that are able to change in response to input from the environment.

pons   The middle structure of three structures in the brainstem. It works with the medulla to organize postural and vital reflexes and with the midbrain to control levels of sleep and arousal.

positron emission tomography   Also known as PET, a method used to research which areas of the brain are active during a certain task. Radioactive dye is injected into the cranial bloodstream and then tracked. The most active areas show the highest levels of radioactivity.

posterior   Directional term meaning "toward the back of the brain." Posterior is the opposite of anterior.

prefrontal cortex   The most anterior part of the frontal lobe; involved in inhibition and other functions of the frontal lobe. It is the most recently developed part of the brain.

primary auditory cortex   Located in the temporal lobe on the edge of the lateral fissure; analyzes sound input from receptors in the ear.

primary motor cortex   Controls directed movements of the body through nerves that travel though the brainstem and spinal cord to the muscles of the body.

primary visual cortex   Located in the occipital lobe; receives signals from the retina (part of the eye) and analyzes visual information to help form a coherent picture of the world we see.

psychiatrists   Medical doctors with special training in the diagnosis and treatment of mental illness.

psychologists   Professionals in the mental health field who have completed a doctoral degree in psychology from an accredited doctoral program and have finished an internship of supervised professional experience.

psychotic   Unable to distinguish reality from imaginary stimuli and inner thoughts from outside voices.

schizophrenia   A neurological disorder marked by social dysfunction and psychotic symptoms that last for at least six months.

sensory areas   Term used to encompass regions of the cortex that receive input from the senses, primarily the visual cortex, the somatic sensory cortex, and the auditory cortex.

sensory neuron   These carry input from sensory receptors all over the body to the brain and spinal cord.

serotonin   Chemical in the brain that regulates emotions. Lack of serotonin can cause depression.

SPECT   Single photon emission computed tomography, used to see how blood flows through the arteries and veins in your brain.

spectrum disorder   A medical or psychiatric condition which can exhibit itself on a spectrum ranging from mild to severe. Examples include bipolar disorder and autism.

spinal cord   The part of the body that contains motor and sensory nerves that carry information between the brain and the body.

SSRIs   Selective serotonin reuptake inhibitors, a commonly prescribed type of anti-depressants used to increase the levels of serotonin in the brain.

sulcus   An inward fold in the surface of the brain's tissue.

superior   Directional term meaning "toward the top of the brain." Superior is the opposite of inferior.

sympathetic system   Part of the autonomic system that controls bodily functions that mediate the "fight or flight" response to stress.

temporal lobe   Located inferior to the lateral fissure; contains the hippocampus and the amygdala.

thalamus   Subcortical structure; part of the diencephalon that acts as a relay center for signals being sent to, from, or within the brain.

tract   A bundle of nerves that are located close to one other and which generally serve a similar purpose.

Resources

Organizations

American Psychiatric Association
www.psych.org

Child and Adolescent Bipolar Foundation
www.bpkids.org

Depression and Bipolar Support Alliance
www.dbsalliance.org

Mental Health America
www.nmha.org

MentalHelp.net
www.mentalhelp.net

National Alliance on Mental Illness
www.nami.org

National Institute of Mental Health
www.nimh.nih.gov

Agencies

Equal Employment Opportunity Commission
www.eeoc.gov

Protection and Advocacy for Individuals with Mental Illness
www.advocacycenter.org/programs/paimi/index.html

Treatment Facilities

Here is a partial list of treatment facilities for bipolar disorder who responded to my inquiries, dual diagnosis and otherwise. These are believed to be some of the best, but the authors cannot be responsible for outcomes, therefore they are just listed without recommendation either way.

Beth Israel Medical Center, New York City
www.bpfamily.org

Caron Foundation, Pennsylvania
www.caron.org

Government information on Bipolar Disorder
Check out the National Mental Health Information Center
www.mentalhealth.samhsa.gov

Hollywood Pavilion, Florida
www.hollywoodpavilion.com

The Meadows, Arizona
www.themeadows.org

New Directions Delaware, Delaware
www.newdirectionsdelaware.org

Rose Hill Center, Michigan
www.rosehillcenter.com

Sierra Tucson, Arizona
www.sierratucson.com

Skyland Trail, Atlanta
www.skylandtrail.org

Support Groups

Depression and Bipolar Support Alliance (DBSA)—Oversees a network of 1,000 support groups nationwide.
www.dbsalliance.org

Mentally Ill Chemically Addicted (MICA)—Holds free support group meetings all over the United States. Your local Mental Health Association can provide the times and dates for your local chapter.

Online Support Groups and Communities

Bipolar World
www.bipolarworld.net

Publications

BP Magazine
www.bphope.com

Books

Akiskal, Hagop S., Norman Sartorius, Mario Maj, and Juan José Lopez-Ibor, eds. *Bipolar Disorder, Vol. 5*. Wiley, 2002

Doidge, Norman. *The Brain That Changes Itself: Stories of Personal Triumph from the Frontiers of Brain Science*. Penguin Group (USA), 2007.

Advocacy Organizations

The following list is a basic guide to organizations that can help protect your rights as a patient and as a person disabled with mental illness.

American Bar Association
Commission on Mental and Physical Disability Law
740 15th Street NW, 9th Floor
Washington, DC 20005
Telephone: 202-662-1570
Fax: 202-662-1032
E-mail: cmpdl@abanet.org
www.abanet.org/disability

American Civil Liberties Union
of the National Capital Area
1400 20th Street NW
Washington, DC 20036
Telephone: 202-457-0800
www.aclu.org

Disability Rights Section
Civil Rights Division
U.S. Department of Justice
950 Pennsylvania Avenue, NW
Washington, DC 20530
Telephone: 1-800-514-0301
Fax: 202-307-1198
(TDD): 1-800-514-0383
www.usdoj.gov/crt/drssec.htm

Judge Bazelon Center for Mental Health Law
1101 15th Street NW, Suite 1212
Washington, DC 20005
Telephone: 202-467-5730
Fax: 202-223-0409
www.bazelon.org

National Alliance on Mental Illness
Colonial Place Three
2107 Wilson Boulevard, Suite 300
Arlington, VA 22201
Telephone: 1-800-950-6264
Fax: 703-524-9094
www.nami.org

National Disability Rights Network
900 2nd Street NE, Suite 211
Washington, DC 20002
Telephone: 202-408-9514
Fax: 202-408-9520
(TDD): 202-408-9521
www.ndrn.org

National Empowerment Center
599 Canal Street
Lawrence, MA 01840
Telephone: 1-800-769-3728
Fax: 978-681-6426
www.power2u.org

National Mental Health Association
2001 N. Beauregard Street, 12th Floor
Alexandria, VA 22311
Telephone: 1-800-969-NMHA (6642)
Fax: 703-684-5968
www.nmha.org

National Mental Health Consumer's Self-Help Clearinghouse
1211 Chestnut Street, Suite 1207
Philadelphia, PA 19107
Telephone: 1-800-553-4539
Fax: 215-636-6312
E-mail: info@mhselfhelp.org
www.mhselfhelp.org

National Rehabilitation Information Center
4200 Forbes Boulevard, Suite 202
Lanham, MD 20706
Telephone: 1-800-346-2742 or 301-459-5900
E-mail: naricinfo@heitechservices.com
www.naric.com

SAMHSA's National Mental Health Information Center
PO Box 42557
Washington, DC 20015
Telephone: 1-800-789-2647
Fax: 240-747-5470
(TDD): 1-866-889-2647
E-mail: nmhic-info@samhsa.hhs.gov
http://mentalhealth.samhsa.gov

Index

triggers, 39
    fatigue, 43-44
    hormones, 40
    illness/injury, 41
    mania, 63-65
    recreational drug use, 42
    stress, 42-43
    trauma, 41
Trileptal (oxcarbazepine), 142

U

underreporting of BP, 3
unipolar depression, 14
An Unquiet Mind, 151

V

valproic acid, 215
visible disability, 191-192
visualization of consequences, 25
vitamins, 83
voluntary commitments (hospitalization), 168-169

W-X

weight issues, 93-94
Winokur, George, 5
withdrawal
    medications, 114
    as red flag, 98
    as suicidal sign, 101
workplace discrimination, 198-199

Y-Z

young persons, 105
    diagnosis difficulties, 107-108
    effect of puberty, 110-111
    importance of sleep, 111
    medications, 111-113
        delayed effects/dependency/withdrawal, 114
        parental advice, 115-116
    preteens, 109-110
    school problems, 116
    statistics, 106-107
    teenagers, 110
    up to 10 years old, 109

zolpidem, 141

Contributors

Rita L. Warner is a biological anthropologist with an interest in evolutionary psychology and cross-cultural psychiatry. Currently, she is pursuing her doctorate at Binghamton University. She holds an M.A. in anthropology and an M.S. in biomedical anthropology and has taught courses in medical anthropology, human variation, Darwinian medicine, and world health-care systems at Binghamton University and Utica College.

Julie A. Fast is the author of *Loving Someone with Bipolar Disorder: Understanding and Helping Your Partner*; *Take Charge of Bipolar Disorder: A Four Step Plan for You and Your Loved Ones to Manage the Illness and Create Lasting Stability*; and *Get it Done When You're Depressed: 50 Strategies for Keeping Your Life on Track*. You can read more about Julie's work at www.juliefast.com.

Patricia C. Friel, M.S., Professional Clinical Counselor and Licensed Independent Chemical Dependency Counselor, has a Master's degree in mental health counseling from Wright State University in Dayton, Ohio. She is the author of *Aspects of Personal Faith: Personality and Religion in Western and Eastern Traditions*.

Bob Anthony is a poet and author. His books can be found on lulu.com.

Jonathan Gransee is a psychologist specializing in substance abuse counseling and mental health evaluations. His website is http://jgevaluations.com.

David F. O'Connell, Ph.D., is a licensed psychologist in Pennsylvania and New Mexico, with 30 years of clinical experience. He has completed all courses and clinical practica for a postdoctoral Master of Science degree in clinical psychopharmacology at Fairleigh Dickinson University. Dr. O'Connell has been board certified with the American Academy of Psychologists Treating Addiction and is listed in the National Register of Health Service Providers in Psychology. His website is www.selfrecovery.co.nr.